eyeglasses
BUYING GUIDE

eyeglasses

BUYING GUIDE

How to Buy Eyeglasses
and Sunglasses—
Pay Less and Get More

MARK AGNEW

Founder and CEO, Eyeglasses.com

Published by Mark Agnew

Printed in the United States of America
First printing 2018

ISBN: 978-1-7326557-0-6 (paperback)

Why This Book Has No Endorsements

Since leaving Wall Street to found Eyeglasses.com, I have been the bad guy. Since 1999, I have been an outsider in the tightly knit eyewear industry where suppliers, eye doctors, and retailers work closely together to keep prices high and consumers ignorant. For almost twenty years I have been working to educate consumers, increase their choices, and reduce their costs in eyewear. It is truly amazing that, today, this book is the first consumer buying guide written to educate consumers about how to buy eyewear.

Optical dispensaries, your optician, and optometrists everywhere love to hate the internet and all internet stores. They believe that the internet is destroying their business (it isn't), and the online stores are taking business away (they aren't). The fact that consumers purchase eyewear only once every two years shows what a poor job optical stores are doing about selling their product and services.

Buying eyeglasses has become difficult, expensive, and unpleasant—not nearly as enjoyable as buying shoes. And consider this: Even though eyewear is more visible than any other piece of clothing, most people have only one pair of glasses.

Here's my suggestion to the industry: If you lower your prices, you will sell more glasses to more people, be successful doing so, and improve people's lives. Alas, old habits die hard, and these professionals would no sooner endorse this book and the information I am about to tell you than stick a needle in their eye.

Yet I persist—providing valuable information in this book and on my company's website at Eyeglasses.com—and offer massive choice where choice is limited and sell at reasonable prices. This book will save you time, money, and hassles in your next purchase of eyeglasses—and for me, that is success in itself.

CONTENTS

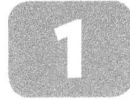

Read This—Before You Buy Another Pair of Glasses

You can watch a YouTube video to help you fix a broken lawn mower or perform a Google search and find helpful instructions on how to buy a car, but you can't easily find information on how to buy the right eyeglasses. Why? Because, quite simply, the optical industry doesn't want you to know.

In an industry whose mission is to help millions see more clearly, the process of buying glasses continues to be murky and dark and cloaked in a cloud of mystery pricing.

In this buying guide, I have pulled back the curtain to reveal the optical industry's dirty little secrets in response to inquiries from my customers who could not find this information anywhere else. It is amazing how little information truly is available to consumers about buying eyeglasses and prescription lenses. Thank you for reading.

Think about the last time you purchased eyeglasses. Did you feel pressured to buy expensive frames? Didn't think you had a choice about lens coatings? Wondered if you had been oversold? Feared you would make the wrong decision about frame shape? Felt compelled to use your vision insurance options but ended up paying way too much for frames anyway?

Information about eyewear is well known to the professionals in eyewear stores, but eyewear stores do not offer books or information about their trade. With this guide, you can make your own choices and be a much more empowered buyer when it comes to these essential features:

- Which frame types are best for my face? (Zero in on the frames that will flatter your face or make a fashion statement by knowing your face shape first and which frames play up your best features.)

- Are expensive frames worth the additional cost? (Yes, but frame quality is not always determined by price. Understand what Made in China really means.)

- Does it matter what the frames are made of? (It does but depends on how active you are and your lifestyle. And sometimes you just want some cheap reading glasses.)

- Should I buy glasses online? (You can if you know a few simple measurements.)

- Which lenses do I want and need? (Making these decisions can often be as bewildering as choosing frames.)

- Do lens coatings make a difference? (Short answer: yes.)

- How can I best use my vision insurance plan? (Guess what? Vision insurance is not insurance at all but a way to charge people without vision insurance more for their glasses. Here's a hack to save big bucks with or without insurance.)

I want to help the millions of Americans who wear glasses and make purchases every year or two but stand in front of eyeglasses frame displays or page through internet screens of designer frames and are asked to make decisions about lenses and coatings and costs without a guide. Just as you might spend a few hours researching how to buy and sell Bitcoin or assemble your fantasy football team roster, spend some time getting smarter about your eyeglasses. If you don't, I guarantee you will pay more and get less when you buy eyewear.

Whether you buy glasses from a retail or discount store or from Eyeglasses.com or from another online eyewear supplier, I just want you to be an informed buyer and know what you're buying and what you'll get.

15 Tips to Save Money at the Eyewear Store

Your eye exam revealed an adjustment to your current eyeglasses prescription. You need new glasses or new lenses in your current frames. Now what?

You sit down with the technician at your local optometry office, optical store, or eyewear chain store. Hold onto your wallet. Or follow these insider tips to save a bundle and get the same high quality you deserve:

1. Be wary of the upsell. Stores are programmed to make you fear basic features and spend more for the add-ons. Learn which add-ons you really want to pay for, before you enter the store. Savings to you: Could be over $100.

2. Eyeglasses lenses are scratch-coated at the factory, so don't pay extra for it. Savings to you: $10 to $35 if you say no to additional costs for scratch coating.

3. Learn the difference between a stock lens and a surfaced lens. If your prescription can be made with a stock lens, the cost to the optician should be half. Savings to you: $30 to $100 if you choose a stock lens.

4. Do you really need a progressive lens? They are convenient, but much more expensive than a single-vision lens (much more about lenses later in this guide). Progressives (lenses used for both distance and reading in the same pair of glasses) are difficult to adjust to. Do not let the optical professional tell you what you need. Savings to you: $100 to $200.

5. So you picked out a frame at a store. Did you check the price

for that frame on the internet? If you find it for lower on the internet, the store owner should match the internet price for it (or buy it yourself on the internet). Savings to you: $20 to $200 if you price match with an internet search and know how to compare frames (I tell you in this guide).

6. If you choose anti-reflective coating, make sure it comes with at least a one-year, anti-scratch warranty (more about coatings later). If it does not come with a warranty, don't pay more than $20 for it. If it comes with a one-year warranty, it is worth around $50 and with a two-year warranty it is worth about $75. Savings to you: $30 to $100.

7. Poly or plastic? Polycarbonate lenses cost the optician about $2 more than regular plastic lenses, but they will upsell it for a lot more. Savings to you: $20 to $40 if you choose plastic lenses, although in some situations (for children, sporting activities, and those who need a stronger prescription) polycarbonate is the better choice.

8. UV protection is automatically included in polycarbonate and high index lenses, so there should be no additional fee. Savings to you: $20 to $30.

9. Rimless glasses are more expensive to make, because they are drill mounted. This requires extra labor for the optician and extra cost for you. Also, only more expensive lens materials can be used. If you avoid rimless eyeglasses, you can save a bundle. Savings to you: $60 to $100 if you choose a frame with a rim.

10. If you need two pairs of prescription glasses, the optician has lower costs on the second pair. Ask your optical professional for a 50% discount on the second pair of lenses. Savings to you: $40 to $200 if you negotiate for two pairs.

11. A single-vision plastic lens is inexpensive to make. The lens itself is about $1.00 and then there is ten minutes of labor to install it. Don't pay more than $50 for it. Savings to you: $20 to $50.

12. Don't cave in to the "blue-light" upsell. Lenses that "block" blue light only block a small proportion of it. You will never be able to notice the difference in a blue-light-blocking lens, and there are no studies to show that a blue-light-blocking lens is actually beneficial in blocking glare. It is not worth the extra fee that is being charged for it. Savings to you: $20 to $50.

13. Use your insurance wisely. Get a price on glasses using your out-of-network benefits (yes, this works because glasses are overpriced to compensate for insurance discounts). Savings to you: For glasses that are priced over $150, you can save anywhere from $25 to $200 depending on your eyewear choices and your plan benefits.

14. You see a lot of advertising around "thin" and "light" lenses, but, in actuality, the thinness of a lens is a function of three factors: (1) your prescription, (2) the size and shape of the lens determined by the frame, and (3) the lens material. If your prescription is under +/- 4.00 sphere, there is no reason to pay more for a lens with an index of refraction higher than 1.60. If your optician is selling you on a "thinner and lighter," more expensive lens, ask them to tell you the difference in thickness and weight between the two options. This could save you $25 to $100 or more, depending on the lens type.

15. Need new lenses only? You don't need an optician to replace lenses in your existing frame. You can find many mail-order services online where you can mail your glasses in, include a new prescription if you have one, and get quality lenses at much lower prices than the optical store. Savings of $50 to $150.

11 Secrets the Eyewear Industry Doesn't Want You to Know

Secret #1:

About twenty-five US states require "Licensed Opticians" to dispense eyewear, and the rest of the states do not. My state—Connecticut—has the most stringent regulations in the entire country. In Connecticut, Licensed Opticians need to enroll in a two-year full-time school or spend four years as an apprentice. Either way, they are then required to take a very difficult exam with a 25% pass rate (according to 2018 test results). This leads to fewer opticians in the regulated states, and higher prices for eyewear in those states. Tip: If you want to pay less, then don't buy eyeglasses in Connecticut or other highly regulated states. Conversely, if you want the highest possible quality of eyeglasses, then buy them in Connecticut, or in another highly regulated state.

Secret #2:

Every eye doctor, optometrist, optician, and optical professional will swear that you are an idiot, moron, and stupid person if you purchase eyewear from the internet. It is true that you cannot get a perfect fitting through the remote sales model of the internet, but in most cases that requirement is exaggerated. Shopping online is definitely not for everyone, but it is not nearly as bad as described by the professionals, who are terrified that the internet will steal their business. Only approximately 3 to 5% of the eyewear industry (by revenue) is conducted on the internet currently—far lower than other fashion categories.

Secret #3:

Eye doctors, optometrists, opticians, and optical professionals may refuse to give you your pupil distance measurement (called the PD), but this is a violation of federal law. The PD is an essential measurement that is part of your custom eyeglasses prescription. It is your information and they are required to disclose it. The only reason they hesitate to give it to you is that they don't want to lose your business and have you buying cheaper glasses on the internet. Don't leave the eye doctor's office without this number written on your prescription.

Secret #4:

Factory prices for an eyeglasses frame range from about $1 to $20 per frame. The cheapest eyeglasses from China cost less than $1, and better-quality Chinese frames cost around $5 each. When you purchase a better designer brand of eyeglasses for $200 to $300, the factory cost was around $20. When you purchase an "unknown" brand for $95, the factory cost was probably around $1, and these frames break more easily. The best value is in the European-made frames that are $150 or less, where you get the best mix of price and sturdiness.

Secret #5:

You can get the same or better-quality frames and lenses through the internet in many cases, but not all cases. Our experience at Eyeglasses.com is that about 90% of people are well served by online eyewear stores. The other 10% of people have diffi-cult-to-fill prescriptions or other requirements that make the internet impractical. Most internet stores sell low-quality, cheap eyeglasses, and if the glasses don't work for your prescription, it is very difficult to talk to a human being about the problem to get a remake of the lenses. Look for an internet store that will answer the phone or respond to email or chat so that if you need help, you know you can get it.

Secret #6:

Lens quality is a function of the doctor's prescription, the lens itself, the optician, and the lens laboratory. All four of these must work together, or your vision will be compromised, and a mistake in any one of these could cause a problem. Making a perfect lens is as much of an art as a science, and sometimes lenses need to be rechecked and remade to get it right. Some optical stores will try to force you to live with sub-par lenses instead of remaking them. If this happens to you, insist on a full refund and go to a different optician.

Secret #7:

Before you give the optician your lens job, check their reviews on Yelp and other online review services. Also ask them about their lens return and redo policy: What happens if your vision is not perfect, will they remake the lenses (the answer should be yes)? How many times will they do that (should be at least once)? What happens if there is a doctor's change (they should redo once or twice)? What happens if you just don't like the glasses and want to return them (they should offer a onetime free redo)? If you don't like the answers to any of these questions, try another optical store.

Secret #8

In general, optometrists write better prescriptions than ophthalmologists, who care more about medical issues than eyeglasses prescriptions. I have seen many more "doctor's changes" from prescriptions written by ophthalmologists than optometrists, so if you have the choice, visit an optometrist for your annual checkup, and he or she will refer you to an ophthalmologist if a medical problem is detected.

Secret #9

Lenses and lens coatings are made under established brand names (Essilor, Zeiss, Pentax, Kodak, Varilux, Crizal, Transitions, Seiko, and many more) and under generic names. Generic lenses are less expensive for the optician to purchase—usually about half the cost of a branded lenses—and generally have lower quality. For single-vision lenses, the quality difference may be minor. But for progressive lenses, the difference in the usability of the lens could be significant. Ask for a branded lens, and if you are quoted a much higher price for it, shop around.

Secret #10

Eye doctors often write on a prescription information like "progressive" or "no-line bifocal" or "high index" or "polycarbonate" or "anti-reflective." People see this and assume that it is "required" by the doctor. However, these are your choices based on your lifestyle that you should make; the terms are not requirements. These are upsell items. In most cases, eye doctors write this information in order to sell a more expensive lens (progressive) or additional coatings (anti-reflective).

Secret #11

Progressive lenses provide much more profit to optical stores than single-vision lenses or bifocals. Many people love the benefits of progressive lenses (one pair for distance, intermediate, and near vision, with no visible line) and are willing and able to "accommodate" their problems (more expensive, fuzzy vision at the sides, which requires you to move your head, possible headaches and dizziness trying to get used to them). Ask the optical store about their return policy if you don't like the progressive lenses and can't get used to them, because some stores will not provide a refund.

10 Reasons Not to Buy Cheap Glasses

Don't be pennywise and pound foolish. In other words, don't be a cheapskate when it comes to your vision. The internet offers many stores and options to purchase cheap eyeglasses. This may be a good option for some people, but you should be aware of the many problems that could crop up with a pair of cheap eyeglasses.

Here's why you don't want to buy cheap eyeglasses:

1. Cheap eyeglasses frames break, usually because of defects or low-quality components at the hinges or nose pads. Then you have to start over with the frames and lenses. This is very inconvenient if you rely on your glasses every day.

2. If cheap frames break, it is usually impossible to get spare parts to fix the frame.

3. Cheap frames look cheap, because they are made with nylon and other low-quality materials.

4. Cheap lenses scratch more easily.

5. Cheap lenses often see their coatings flake and discolor over time.

6. Cheap lenses have more distortions in the plastic, making it harder to see through.

7. Cheap lenses may not be made perfectly for your prescription and your face.

8. Cheap progressive lenses have a smaller viewing area, making them more uncomfortable to use.

9. Cheap optical stores offer poor quality customer service—or no service at all.

10. Cheap eyewear stores often charge restocking fees, or don't accept returns at all.

Have I convinced you that you need to understand the eyewear business to get the right frames and lenses for your vision correction, that prices vary (and you should not overpay for quality), and that you do have control of this decision as an empowered patient? Let's get down to the nitty gritty about glasses.

2

How to Choose the Most Flattering Eyeglasses Frames for Your Face

How many magazine articles or blogs have you read that claim to help you assess just the right frame shape and color that will flatter your face? It's not magic. Like clothing, some frames just look better or feel better or highlight your best assets or play down your other assets, but the bottom line with frames is this: Choose a frame that you like, that fits, and that helps you see better.

DETERMINE YOUR FACE SHAPE

Frame shapes can be used to accentuate or de-accentuate your facial features, depending on how you choose to express your personality. For example, if your face is basically round, round glasses would reinforce that look, and rectangular glasses would reduce the roundness of your face.

For those who wish to know the current thinking in the optical community on face shapes and frames, let me explain.

The shape of your face can be complemented by the shape of your glasses. To understand how glasses shapes can affect your face, begin by understanding the fundamentals of face shape and proportion because this is the first step in selecting glasses that help you look your best. While most faces are a combination of shapes and angles, here are six basic face shapes and guidelines for which types of frames work for each.

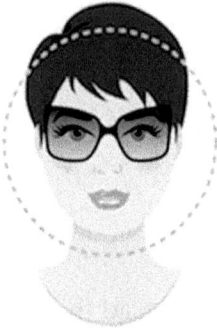

Round Face

A round face shape has curvilinear lines with the width and length in the same proportions and no angles. Your goal is to make your face appear longer and thinner. Look for angular, narrow frames that will lengthen the face; high or mid-height temples, which help create a longer profile; a clear bridge that widens the eyes; colored temples to add width; and glasses frames that are wider than they are deep, such as an octagonal shape.

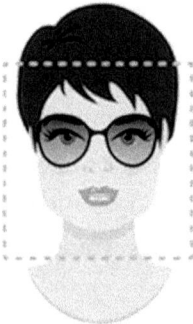

Square Face

A square face shape is characterized by a strong jaw line and a broad forehead—the face width and length are in the same proportions. Your goal should be to make your face look longer and soften the angles. Look for curvilinear, narrow-style glasses that soften facial angles; frames that are wider than the widest part of the face; eyeglasses that have more width than depth; narrow oval glasses are an excellent choice.

Oval Face

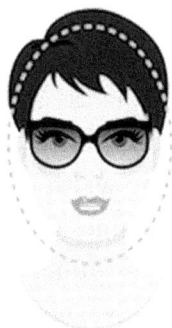

The oval face shape is considered to be the ideal shape because of its balanced proportions. The oval face is neither round nor angular. Your goal should be to keep the oval's natural balance. Look for glasses frames that are as wide as, or wider than, the broadest part of your face. Look for almond or walnut-shaped frames that are neither too deep nor too narrow so that they do not upset facial balance.

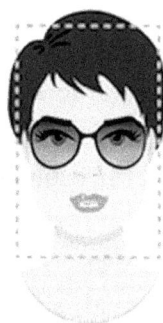

Oblong Face

The oblong or rectangular face shape is longer than it is wide and is characterized by a long, straight cheek line and sometimes a longer nose. Your goal should be to make your face appear shorter and more balanced. Look for glasses frames that have top-to-bottom depth such as rounder panto or P-3 shapes (more about this later); decorative or contrasting temples that can add width to the face; and a low bridge to shorten the nose.

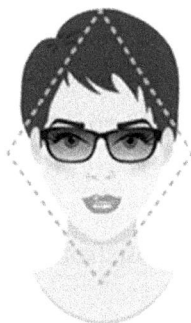

Diamond Face

Diamond-shaped faces are narrow at the eyeline and the jawline. Cheekbones are frequently high and dramatic. The diamond is the rarest face shape. Your goal should be to highlight your eyes and bring out the cheekbones. Look for frames that have detailing or distinctive brow lines. Rimless frames, ovals, or cat-eyes are all excellent choices.

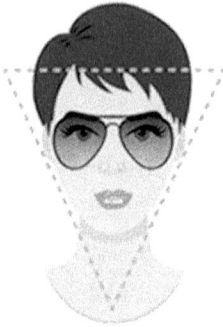

Base-Up Triangle Face

The base-up triangle face shape has a very wide top third and small bottom third. Your goal should be to minimize the width of the top half of the face. Look for frames that are wider at the bottom half of the frame. Very light colored materials are effective, and rimless styles are an excellent choice.

NOW CHOOSE A FRAME SHAPE

There are thousands of subtle differences among frame shapes and sizes. The shape and size of the frame usually depends on your choice, based on what you think looks good on your face. Only in a few cases does the prescription restrict the shape and size of an eyeglasses frame.

Whether a frame is basically rectangular or oval is in the eye of the beholder. There are thousands of gradations and subtleties. In the end it really doesn't matter what you call a frame's shape. What is important is whether you like it on your face or not.

Rectangular frames are somewhat squared off in their appearance. Modified rectangles are rectangles with softened corners. Oval frames have curves rather than lines in the outline. Most designer eyewear frames have either round or oval shapes.

Here are the basic shapes of frames you will choose from in the optical shop or online:

Round

One of the most classic (but hard to find) frame shapes is the round frame. Round frames are perfectly round. John Lennon popularized these frames.

The round frame is the most popular of all time.

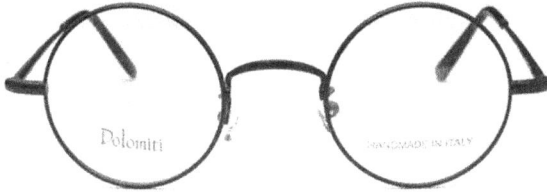

Panto

The panto or P-3 frame shape gets its name from the eyewear manufacturers, and it refers to a classic style that falls between oval and round. The top of the frame is round and flattish, and the bottom of the frame is round but slightly pointed.

The panto shape is the most enduring and popular frame

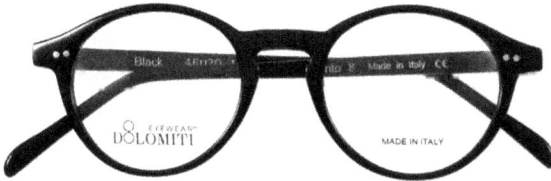

Aviator

The aviator frame shape is named after WWII aviators who wore frames with a distinctive shape. Each eye has a teardrop shape, with a diagonal cut from the nose down to the cheeks.

Aviator style was made popular by pilots in WWII

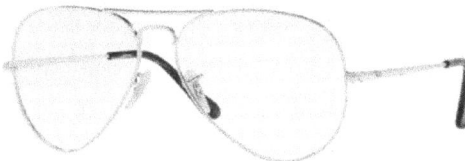

Cat-eye

Cat-eye frames are slightly pointed at the sides by the ears. The frame is elongated. These were very popular in the 1950s and 1960s, and the retro look is coming back.

Cat-eye shaped frames, popular in the 1950s, are making a comeback

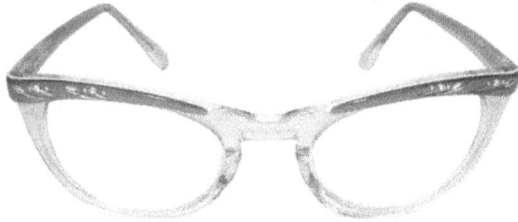

Half-eye

Half-eye frames are designed to sit lower on the wearer's nose, allowing the wearer to look over the top of the lens easily. Half-eye frames are designed to be used as reading glasses so the reader can look down to read but can see in the distance when looking straight ahead without the glasses interfering with the line of sight.

The half-eye frame sits low on your face so you ca look over the top or down to read

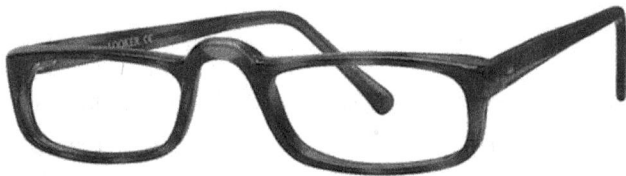

Frame coloring works the same way as frame shapes. You choose the frame color to either match or contrast with skin and hair tone, eye color, jewelry, and clothing colors. The degree to which you match or contrast will contribute to the expression of your personality and your look.

TIME TO PICK A FRAME TYPE

The optical industry groups frames into three basic frame types: full frame, half-rimless frame, and rimless frame.

Full Frames

A full glasses frame has a rim that completely encircles the lens.

Half-Rimless Frames

A half-rimless frame design has a rim over the top half of the lens (and sometimes just on the bottom half). In most cases the bottom part of the lens is held in place by a nylon cord, but some frames are drill mounted so the cord is not necessary. The frame on a half-rimless frame is most commonly on the top of the lens, and people choose it for style reasons. Some reading glasses designs are rimless on the top, because it is easier to look over the top of the lens.

A half-rimless frame has a rim just around the top

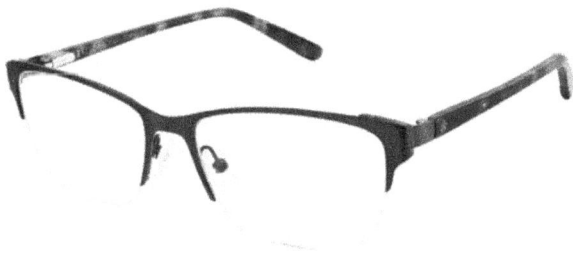

Rimless Frames

Rimless glasses frames have no frame at all around the lens. Rimless eyeglasses come in three pieces (two temples and the nose part). The lenses are actually part of the structure of the frame, so it is important to only use high index, polycarbonate, or Trivex lens material on rimless glasses (more on materials used to make lenses coming up soon).

Mounting lenses into rimless frames is tricky and requires a skilled and experienced technician. Each lens must be drilled perfectly so that the frame fits snugly into the lens. Poorly mounted rimless frames will begin to rattle and can eventually crack the lens.

A rimless frame has no frame around the lenses

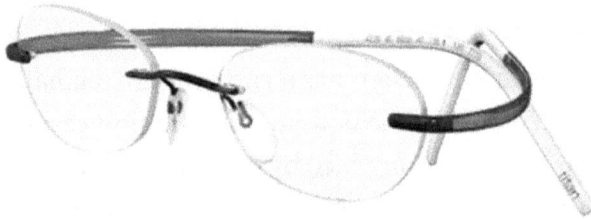

Rimless frames have been around for years (you've seen them on people in old photos, I mean really old photos, at least 100 years old), but this style has recently been rediscovered and is now featured by many of the top designer eyewear brands.

Rimless eyeglasses have less frame material, and no frame around the rim of the lens, so the glasses seem to float on the face. Rimless glasses, of all the frame designs, reveal the greatest amount of your face. The light lines and contours of rimless glasses add a delicacy, grace, and refined quality that regular frames cannot provide.

Rimless glasses are ultralight and very comfortable to wear. The really light rimless titanium glasses, like the Silhouette brand rimless eyeglasses, are feather light and a real pleasure to wear, especially if you are used to wearing heavy glasses. Not only are they light, but they tend to stay in one place better than regular glasses.

Rimless frames are available in many different shapes, sizes, colors, and styles. You can choose among rimless frames made of plastic, metal, or titanium. Some are made with regular hinges, with spring hinges, or with no hinges. Rimless glasses come with nose pads, and without nose pads (called a saddle bridge). In general, rimless frames cost a little more than their rimmed counterparts because it is more complicated to mount the lenses into rimless glasses.

Rimless glasses vary in the construction of the frame and how it is attached to the lenses. Double-drilled frames are much less likely to begin rattling and to loosen, but it is a more technically difficult job to mount the glasses, so you need to be sure the optical professional doing the mounting has had a lot of experience. Most rimless glasses do not have a double-drilled construction. Instead, they have a notched construction, which is easier for the optical professional to make, but is more likely to loosen up over time.

If you don't know what you're looking at when considering frames, ask the optical professional or read the online description (or ask customer service).

WHAT MATERIALS ARE FRAMES MADE OF (AND DOES IT MATTER)?

Eyeglasses frames are made out of many different composite materials and formulas, but the basic groupings are metal and plastic. In plastics, zyl is the most common although lower quality plastics are used in the cheaper frames. Nylon is often used in sport sunglasses due to its impact resistance and flexibility. Among the metals, monel is most common, followed by titanium, stainless steel, nickel silver, alpaca, and aluminum.

Let's look at the pluses and minuses of the various frame materials:

Zyl

Zyl is a short name for the material cellulose acetate, which is made of wood flakes, cottonseed fibers, stabilizers, and plasticizers (well, you asked). Zyl is the most common plastic frame material because it can assume a large array of colors, textures, and patterns.

Temples and frame fronts can be cut from blocks of zyl extruded as a sheet of block acetate. Or granular zyl can be liquefied and then injection molded. Block-cut zyl is stronger and more stable, while injection molded zyl is less stable and less expensive. You may not know how the frames were manufactured, but just know about the material itself.

With daily use in warm temperatures, zyl can shift and lose its form. Sometimes metal cores are added in the temples in order to strengthen and stabilize the frame. If zyl frames reach a temperature over 160 degrees Fahrenheit, the plasticizers could rise to the surface of the frame, turning areas of the frame a milky white color (a good reason not to leave glasses tossed on the dashboard in summer). In addition, body oils, perspiration, ultraviolet radiation, and cosmetics can also damage the material.

The best quality designer frames are made with Italian Mazzuccheli zyl. Mazzuccheli now has factories in Italy and China, with the best quality and newest design materials coming from the Italian plants. All Mazzuccheli zyl is made in sheets, which are then cut in the eyewear factories.

A zyl frame is made of cellulose acetate, a common material for eyewear

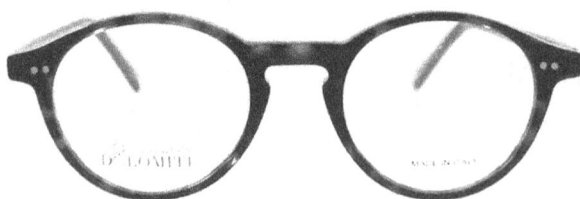

Monel

Monel is composed of about two-thirds nickel and one-third copper. This is a highly ductile alloy, which means it can be hammered into a variety of different shapes without losing strength. It resists stress well and is often used to stabilize frame bridges (bridges on your nose, not a bridge over a river) and end pieces. Monel colors well, is corrosion resistant, and durable. If you have an allergy to some metals, it is usually the nickel in the metal that causes allergic reactions. People with an allergic sensitivity should use frames made entirely of titanium, stainless steel, aluminum, or cellulose acetate (plastic).

Frames made of monel are common for eyewear

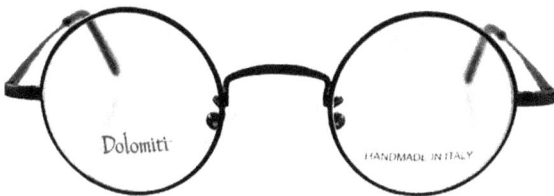

Dolomiti

HANDMADE IN ITALY

Titanium

Titanium is a more expensive metal composite used in frames and known for its beneficial qualities of strength, lightness, and flexibility. Titanium will not rust, making it a very popular and relatively new material for frames. Titanium's strength allows it to be made thin, but it is hard to solder or weld and is expensive. One downside is that titanium is difficult to color so titanium frames usually come in a very restricted range of frame colors.

Titanium frames are light and flexible. also hypo-allergenic. and often used for rimless designs

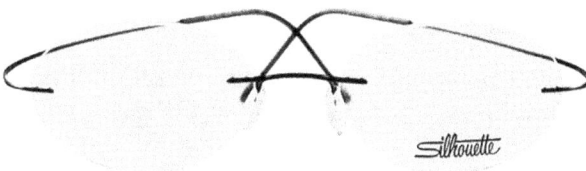

Silhouette

Eyeglasses frames that are 100% titanium are also hypo-allergenic. In other words, they do not contain any nickel, which causes allergic reactions in some people. If you're prone to be allergic to other substances such as plastics, stainless, and whatever else might be causing irritation, the 100% titanium frames are a good choice for you. Many designer brands use titanium in some part of their collection.

Stainless Steel

Stainless steel is composed mostly of iron, with a mixture of nickel, manganese, and chromium. Stainless steel is highly lustrous and makes a good thin and sturdy frame with strong corrosion resistance. Although it is hard to make frames with stainless steel due to soldering and welding difficulties, stainless steel temples are especially springy.

Stainless steel frames are light and also hypo-allergenic

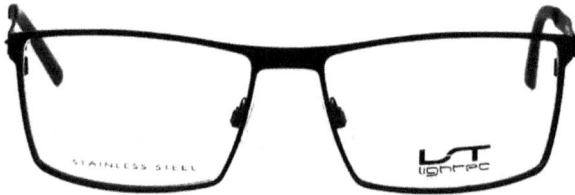

Nylon

Nylon is virtually unbreakable, so it is often chosen for sports and safety applications. Nylon is lightweight and flexible, but can only accept opaque colors.

Nickel Silver, Alpaca, and German Silver

Sometimes called alpaca or German silver, nickel silver is rigid compared to other more malleable metals. Nickel silvers contain more than 50% copper, 25% nickel, and the rest zinc (in fact, no silver at all). Copper adds pliability, zinc adds strength, and nickel gives it its namesake color, a whitish appearance, because when the nickel content exceeds 12%, the copper color no longer shows through. Although the metal is lustrous, its brittleness makes it a poor choice for slender frame fronts and nose pads. Thus, it is better designed for use in hinges, end pieces, bridges, and ornamental trims, as well as an inner core for temples.

Aluminum

Aluminum is cut from a block and is lightweight and low in density. This makes the material strong, yet light enough to use for thick fashion designs. Aluminum can accept a variety of colors, and chemical anodizing is sometimes used to create black, brown, and gold colors. Because aluminum cannot be easily welded or soldered, end pieces, hinges, and nose pads must be fastened with rivets or screws, which increases the chance that those pieces might fall out causing the frame to fail. This greatly limits the design possibilities.

Aluminum is also very stiff, which limits its versatility. However, the lightness and stiffness of aluminum in some eyeglasses designs offers great advantages. For example, for metal frames that are thicker in design, and larger in design, aluminum is the toughest material and can accommodate the thickest and heaviest lenses. Aluminum frames last a long time and can take a lot of abuse compared to plastic frames or thin metal frames.

Flexible Memory Metal

Flexon is a trade name for one company's flexible eyewear frame material. Another big name is TitanFlex. Flexible frames with what's known as memory metal are available in many compositions, but the goal is always the same. This kind of material is used to reduce breakage. The material is normally found in the shaft of the temple and in the bridge, and it allows these areas to endure tremendous twisting without breakage or permanent distortion of the frames shape.

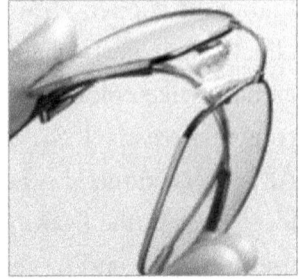

Flexible frame materials are harder to break

These flexible frames are a perfect solution from fit (won't stretch) to finish (lots of colors and shapes are available) and for their strength and flexibility.

If you don't know what a frame is made of, certainly ask.

BLUEPRINT FOR A FRAME AND ITS PARTS

Eyeglasses frames have several components and the names of the different frame parts are useful to learn. Frames have two basic parts: the frame front that holds the lenses, and the temples that hold the frame from falling off your face. It's that simple.

A typical eyeglasses frame and its key parts

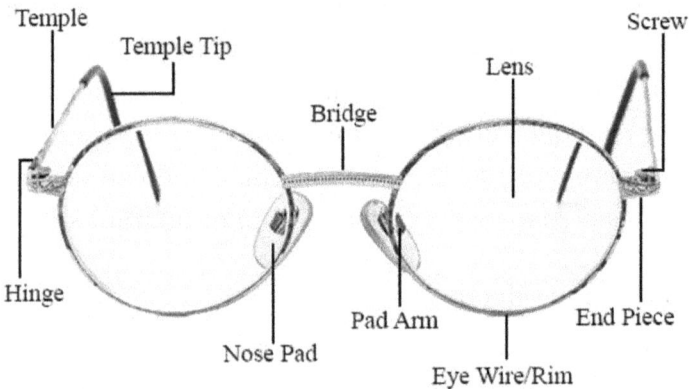

The frame front is composed of two eyepieces connected by the bridge. The eyepieces hold the lenses and connect to the temples by hinges, and the bridge is the part over your nose. Usually, there is just one piece of material connecting the two eyepieces, called a single bridge construction. Some, especially larger, frames have a double-bridge for extra support, with two pieces of material connecting the two eyepieces.

The eyepieces on a full frame completely encircle the lens. On metal frames, the eyepiece is held together with a screw that is removed when the lenses are installed, and then replaced. On plastic frames, the eyepiece is heated until it expands, the lens is snapped into position, and the frame cools and contracts snugly around the lens.

On half-rimless frames, the lens in held in place by a nylon cord called the eye wire that attaches to the frame in two places. The rim of a pair of eyeglasses is the part of the frame eyepiece that holds the lens in place. The rim can completely encircle a lens in the case of full frames, or partially hold the frame in the case of semi-rimless frames, or there can be no rim at all in the case of rimless frames.

On the outer edge of each eyepiece some material extends out beyond the shape of the lens. This is called the end piece, and connected to it is the hinge, which holds the temples to the frame front. End pieces can be designed larger so that a larger person can wear a somewhat smaller lens without the frame pinching the sides of the head.

Many eyeglasses frames, most commonly metal frames, have nose pads attached to the inside of the bridge. Nose pads are normally made of a plastic or silicone and help to comfortably rest the frame on your nose. Nose pads can be adjusted to accommodate an individual's nasal structure, as well as the proper positioning of the lenses in front of your nose.

Nose pads are attached to pad arms, which are welded to the frame front. Nose pad arms are made of a malleable metal so that they can be adjusted (bent) during a fitting. This metal is then welded on to the frame front, which could be made of titanium, monel, stainless, or other materials.

Occasionally these weld points weaken and the pad arms break off the frame there. Nose pads are attached either by a screw (screw-in nose pads), or they are push-in nose pads, which require no screw. Most nose pads are designed this way so that the nose pads can be replaced when they wear out. Pad arms are always made out of malleable metal so they can be adjusted, even on titanium or aluminum frames.

Plastic eyewear frames and some metal frames do not have nose pads; they have a saddle bridge construction instead. This term refers to a style of bridge in which the arched portion of the bridge lies directly on the bridge of the wearer's nose. Saddle bridges are more common with plastic frames than with metal frames. Metal frames with saddle bridges do not have nose pads.

Many different types of frame temples connect and hold the frame front to the wearer's head behind and below the ears. The most common is the skull temple, with the long straight shaft that is bent with a 45-degree angle at the top of the ear near the end of the temple, which is called the temple tip. The shaft is the straight part that extends from the connection point at the frame front to the bend in the temple. Library temples are straight all-shaft temples with no bend in them.

Most eyeglasses frame temples have temple tips that are malleable so that they can be changed (bent) to adjust the fit of the glasses. Frames that are made of titanium, aluminum, and stainless often have a different type of metal welded on to the temple tips. Temple tips are usually coated with a plastic material that is designed to give and adjust to the metal if the metal is bent during an adjustment. These plastic temple tip covers can become worn out, and on some frames they are designed to be replaced.

Cable temples refers to curly temple tips, which curl behind your ears. Cable temples hold glasses in place better and are a good choice for people in active situations and for children. However, cable temples are not easy to adjust, and if they pinch your ear, it is difficult to adjust the temples because the metal is not designed to be adjusted easily.

Eyeglasses frame hinges are used to connect the temples to the front of the frame, while allowing the temple to fold flat against the frame. Most frames use external hinges, which are mounted on the inside of the temple shaft. Internal hinges are buried inside the shaft of the temple, hiding the mechanism from view. Hinges are a small but important component in the overall quality of your frame.

If the hinge is not mounted on the frame properly, it will disengage, which leads to a difficult (or impossible) repair job. Low-quality hinges will wear out, or the screw will pop out and get lost. Poor quality hinges can start to rattle and be floppy. Wrap some duct tape around the broken hinge for a quick repair (just kidding).

Good quality hinges have a smooth and consistent action that does not wear over time, with friction that is consistent throughout the entire range of motion. We still find that the best quality hinges are made in Germany. You can find these in European and Chinese frames and in most better-quality frames. Unfortunately, it is difficult to find out from the manufacturers which hinges they use in a particular frame.

A spring hinge is mounted on the temple shaft and allows for spring action. Spring action hinges can bend beyond the limit of normal hinges, and this type of design can limit breakage of the frame under stress. Spring action hinges also help to keep frames properly aligned. Spring hinges are found on both external and internal hinges.

Hinge-less frames use a springy material, usually titanium, for the temples. The springiness of the temples lightly pinches your head to hold the glasses in place. This system results in a lighter weight pair of glasses, fewer components that could break, and a sleek design.

By now you are probably holding your current glasses and examining the hinges, the temples, the rims, and nose pads, right? You probably never paid attention to the little parts and pieces unless something went wrong and you had to find a teeny-tiny screwdriver and attempt a repair. Now you know what can go wrong, what can break, which materials are more durable, and why you want to pay attention to these features next time you're selecting eyeglasses frames.

SIZE MATTERS (SORT OF) IN EYEGLASSES FRAMES

Frame size is first and foremost a fashion decision. The size of an eyeglasses frame is not that critically important—believe it or not—for fitting eyeglasses because eyeglasses are designed so that the temples, nose pads, and bridge can be adjusted to fit properly. Let me help you find the right size of glasses that you want and understand how to measure frame size.

For any person, there is no one right size of glasses. Your face can accommodate a wide variety of glasses sizes and most glasses will work for most people. In order to understand why this is true, you need to look at what size means: size in glasses is a far different concept than size in shoes or clothing. As a result, you should focus most on how the glasses look on your face. When you find glasses that look good, in most cases the glasses can be adjusted to fit your face.

The rule of thumb is that the total width of the glasses front all the way across, including the end pieces, should be similar to the width of your head. This will allow for the optimum proportion of the glasses to your head and for the best comfort.

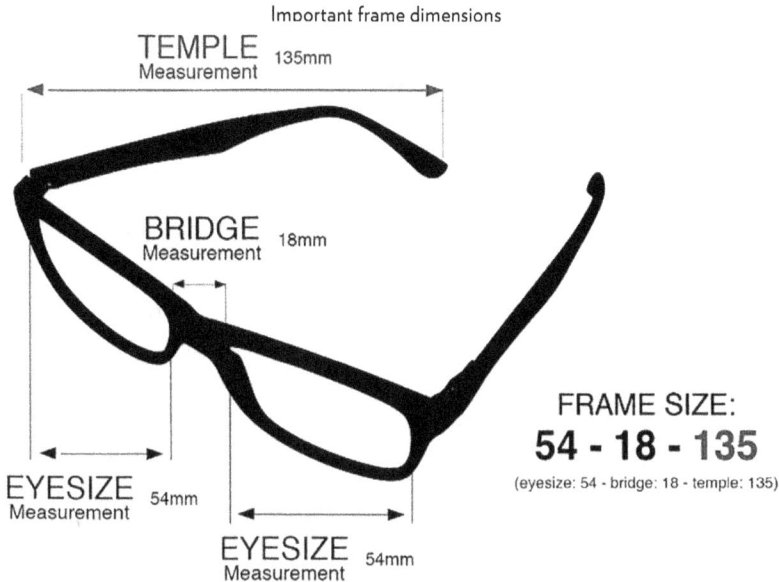

Important frame dimensions

TEMPLE Measurement 135mm

BRIDGE Measurement 18mm

FRAME SIZE:
54 - 18 - 135
(eyesize: 54 - bridge: 18 - temple: 135)

EYESIZE Measurement 54mm

EYESIZE Measurement 54mm

Glasses frames have four basic measurements: the eye, bridge, temple, and **B** measurements.

- The eye size refers to the horizontal width in millimeters of one of the lenses. The measurement is taken from the inside of one side of the frame to the inside of the other side of the frame. The lens is measured from its furthest point, where it would intersect with a vertical line.

- The bridge measurement is the distance in millimeters between the two lenses. It is measured between the two closest points of the two lenses.

- The temple length is measured along the length of the temple, from one end to the other, including the bend. Many frames are constructed with an end piece that extends from the frame front back along the line of the temple. This backward extension of the end piece could be as little as 2 mm, or as much as 15 mm. When the end piece extends farther back, the temple length tends to be smaller to compensate. As a result, if you are accustomed to a 145 mm temple length, a 135 mm temple could work perfectly for you if your new frame has an end piece that extends back 10 mm. This is also the case with many sunglasses with a wrap design. The wrap has the effect of bringing the frame front back toward the ears, thereby requiring a shorter temple length to compensate.

- The B measurement refers to the vertical height of an eyeglasses lens and is measured from the tip to the bottom of the lens aperture of the frame. The measurements are taken from a horizontal line intersecting with the top of the lens, to the horizontal line intersecting with the bottom edge of the lens. The B measurement is only important when making progressive or multifocal lenses.

Reading Your Frame Size

Most glasses frames have some size information printed on the inside of the frame, although the lettering can be worn away with use. To find all the lettering, you must look on the inside of both temples and on the inside of the bridge. The numbers usually look something like this:

GU125 635 50 17 135.

For this frame, it means that the model number is GU125, color number 635, with size 50-17-135. In this case, the brand Guess is abbreviated GU, followed by the model number of the frame. The eye size (50) is followed by bridge size (17), sometimes with a small square box in between. The temple length (135) could be printed after the eye and bridge sizes, or elsewhere.

Other letters and numbers could refer to the color of the frame. The B measurement is never written on the frame. And just when you thought you had all the mystery numbers decoded, consider this. These sizes do not give you all the information that you need to know for sure how big the glasses frame is. To know truly how big the frame is—meaning how will it look on your face—you must determine the total frame width.

The total frame width includes the end pieces, and the end pieces are never measured and specified. The end piece refers to the width of the frame from the edge of the lens out to the edge of the frame where the temples are connected to the frame front. On the product pages of online stores you may see in the frame details the "screw to screw" measurement, which tells how wide the frame actually is.

Now, once you have determined the total frame width, you can use that value to compare to your current glasses, or you can hold a ruler up to your face to get an idea how well the frame will line up with the sides of your head. End pieces vary in size from 3 mm to 15 mm each, which adds up to 6 mm to 30 mm of the total frame width. The rule of thumb is that end pieces add up to about 10% of the total frame width.

There are some cases where a large glasses frame on a small head could look oversized, and a small glasses frame on a large person may hurt (as the temples persistently dig into the sides of your head). But even in extreme situations, you choose frames first on how they look on your face.

An Easier Way

Now, forget everything I just said about measuring and calculating. The easiest and fastest way to find the right size glasses for you is to use your current glasses as a benchmark.

Once you know the size of your current glasses by looking on the inside of the temple (or call your optical store to read you the size from your record), you have a frame of reference, so to speak, for a new pair of glasses.

If the lettering has worn off or is too small for you to see even with a magnifying glass, you can measure your glasses with a millimeter ruler. The eye size is measured from one side of the lens to the other, horizontally, at the widest points. The bridge size is the distance between the lenses at the closest point. The temple size is measured from the tip to the hinge, including the bend.

Let's say for example that your glasses have this size: 50-20-145. You can now use the internet to search for eyeglasses with a similar size. When you do the search, search the eye size range 49-51, and search the bridge range 18-22, and do not search the temple size. Temple size is really not important except in very special cases. Searching a range of sizes is important because it vastly increases the number of results you will get, and also the difference in sizes will be almost unnoticeable compared to your current eyeglasses.

A frame model is usually available in just one size, meaning one combination of eye, bridge, and temple lengths. Occasionally a frame may have more than one size: for example, 50-17-135 B40, and 52-17-135 B42, and 54-18-140 B43. You cannot mix and match the measurements, you must take the whole set of measurements for a given frame and you cannot choose a different collection of measurements. For some manufacturers, if a frame model has more than one available temple length, you may be able to swap temples, but you must contact the company's customer service department to find out if this is possible for the frame you want.

FRAME QUALITY—NOT ALWAYS DETERMINED BY PRICE (AND WHY "MADE IN CHINA" IS NO JOKE)

Determining glasses frame quality is quite difficult, even for an eyewear industry professional. The most reliable determinant of the quality of a pair of glasses frames is the feel of them in your hand. Do they rattle (bad)? Does the temple fit well at the hinge (good)? When you exercise the hinges, do they move smoothly and with the same friction throughout the bend (good)?

A better-quality frame has a higher level of machined perfection, so that the better-quality parts fit together well. Just because a designer frame has a brand affiliation, it does not mean that the glasses frame is of high quality.

Today, about 90% of all eyeglasses are made in China. All of the major Italian glasses frame companies have moved the majority of their production to China. Many of the eyeglasses that are made in China are then shipped to Europe where a minimal amount of assembly or finishing work is done so that the glasses frames can receive the Made in Europe designation. Some popular frames may be produced first in Europe, and later production is moved to China.

Some designers, like Alain Mikli, Lafont, and Silhouette and a few others, make their glasses frames completely in Europe. Brands like Armani, Gucci, and other big fashion houses are mostly made in China, and then finished in Europe. This is not to say that all China eyewear is of inferior quality. The large European eyewear companies have been working closely with Chinese factories for years and the quality could be good.

Glasses frames, as I have explained, are a composite of many different parts. Eyewear manufacturers source parts from all around the world and can assemble glasses frames in different places as well. A plastic glasses frame is composed of the plastic frame front, plastic temples (with wire running through part of the shaft), and hinges. Metal glasses are composed of the metal frame front, metal in the temples, plastic jackets to cover the temples, hinges, frame front, nose pads, and nose pad arms.

Using German hinges and Italian Mazzucchelli zyl (the best) results in an excellent quality European glasses frame. This same frame model could use Mazzucchelli zyl from China (same company, different factory), and Chinese hinges, and be assembled in a Chinese factory. The Chinese frame would be very difficult to differentiate from the original, except that it should be designated Made in China.

Now, let's say that this same frame model used Mazzucchelli zyl from China and Chinese hinges, but was assembled in Italy. It would be called Italian eyewear, Made in Italy. Most European eyewear today (except for a few high-end brands) that is made in Europe is made mostly of Chinese components. Now you know.

Hinges are a small but important component in the overall quality of your glasses frame. We still find that the best quality hinges are made in Germany. You can find these in European and Chinese frames, and in most better-quality frames. Unfortunately, it is difficult to find out from the manufacturers, as I have emphasized, which hinges they use in a particular frame.

For tips on ordering frames online with prescription lenses or sending in your current frames for replacement lenses, see the chapter on how to buy glasses online.

3

Which Lenses Are Right for You?

Now that you have your frames picked out, it's a simple matter of handing your eyeglasses prescription to the optical technician, and depending on the type of store, you may wait an hour or several days for your lenses to be crafted and inserted into the frames you've chosen.

Oh, not so fast.

First, you will be asked several questions about the type of lenses you want and need. Of course, you don't know exactly, because the optical industry has not educated you. You may end up being upsold on several features of lenses you don't want or need and feeling sticker shock when all the add-ons are added up.

Here's what you need to know to make an informed choice about your eyeglasses lenses.

SINGLE-VISION, BIFOCAL, TRIFOCAL, OR PROGRESSIVE?

Your eyes may need vision correction only for distance, only for reading, or for both. If you need correction only for distance vision, then you just need single-vision lenses in your prescription glasses. With single-vision lenses, you can look through all areas of the lens and see clearly.

If you need vision correction only for reading and you do not have astigmatism, then you can buy nonprescription glasses for reading (and please see the extensive section about reading glasses further on in this book, especially if you buy reading glasses at the drugstore). If you do have astigmatism, you need prescription reading glasses. In either case, these are still considered single-vision lenses.

The phrase computer glasses refers to any pair of eyeglasses with lenses that have a focal length set at arm's length. These too are called single-vision lenses. Measure the average distance from your face to your computer screen and give that measurement to your eye doctor. The eye doctor will then prescribe an intermediate (arm's length) prescription power to be used in the lenses.

Keep these glasses at your computer for use when you're online. You won't find them helpful for distance vision or reading. And opt for the anti-reflective coating because it helps to reduce the glare from the computer screen (more about coatings coming up).

If you need vision correction for both distance and reading, then you can use two pairs of prescription eyeglasses and alternate, depending on what you need to see. People do this all the time by carrying one set of glasses for reading in a pocket or purse or scattered about the house (and seem to be endlessly saying, "Where did I leave my reading glasses?"). Some wear their reading glasses around their necks on various decorated or plain cords where they don't get lost but can feel annoying.

Or you can choose multifocal lenses (progressive, bifocal lenses, trifocal lenses). Multifocal lenses divide the lens so that part of the lens is for reading (the bottom part) and part of the lens is for distance vision. Bifocal (two areas) and trifocal (three areas) lenses have visible lines that separate the different areas of the lens. Progressive lenses are sometimes called no-line bifocals, but are actually trifocal lenses without the visible lines.

Bifocal lenses have been around for decades. Until the introduction of progressive lenses in the 1990s, bifocal lenses were used by everyone who wanted the convenience of near and far vision correction in the same pair of eyeglasses.

Prescription eyeglasses with progressive lenses were developed because many people wanted the convenience of not having to change their prescription eyeglasses to read, but they did not like other people to see the visible line in the bifocals. Progressive lenses do have another benefit, however, which is that you feel a smooth transition when you move your eyes from distance objects to close-up objects. With a lined bifocal, the transition between viewing areas can be somewhat uncomfortable.

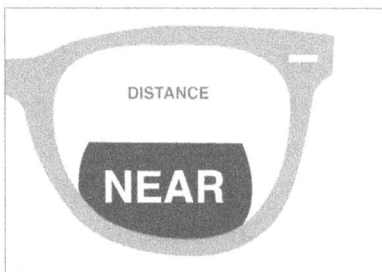

Bifocal lens design has a visible line and one reading area

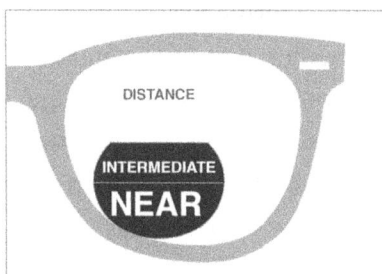

Trifocal lens design has a visible line and two reading areas

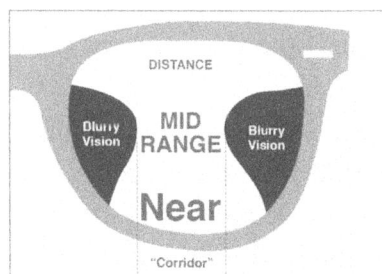

Progressive lens design does not have a visible line

So progressive lenses offer the convenience of multifocals without the visible line. However, progressive lenses are much harder to use and to adapt to than bifocal or trifocal prescription eyeglasses, and they are much more expensive. In order to create a no-line progressive lens, there are two large areas of the lens that you cannot see through. Imagine what an hourglass looks like. This is the shape of the area of the progressive lens that you can see through. Objects seen through the areas of the lens to the left and right of the narrow middle section will be distorted and you cannot see anything there.

The bulge areas at the bottom and top of the lens are for near and distance vision, and the thinner corridor connecting them is for intermediate distances. On either side of the narrow portion of the hourglass, objects will appear distorted. In general, more expensive progressive lenses like Vari-lux have a wider corridor, and less expensive lenses have a narrower corridor that can restrict the viewing area con-siderably.

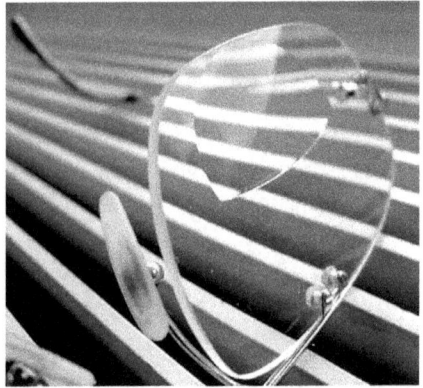

On smaller lens sizes, it is necessary to slice off a portion of the bottom (reading section) of the lens in order to install the lens in the frame. As a result, the smaller the frame size, the smaller will be the reading portion of the lens. If you want to try progressive lenses, be sure to choose a frame size that will work the best.

In order to use progressive prescription glasses, you must learn to move your head to see things; you cannot just move your eyes because you will be looking through a blurry part of the lens. This is called adapting to the lens. Most people can adapt within a month, but some people never adapt. It is common to experience dizziness and headaches during the time that you are adapting. Getting accus-tomed to progressive prescription glasses can be difficult, and you must have proper instruction by an eyecare professional.

Sometimes, people who try progressive prescription glasses have a difficult time learning to look through the appropriate portion of the lens at the right time. Often a simple fitting adjustment to your prescription eyewear by your local optical professional can make all the difference.

NO MORE COKE BOTTLE GLASSES: CHOOSE LENS TYPES

Once you have determined the best lens type for your vision, lifestyle, preferences, and budget, you can then choose the lens material. There are three basic types of lens material for prescription eye glasses:

- Hard resin plastic

- Polycarbonate plastic

- High index plastic

Hard resin lenses are good for most people.

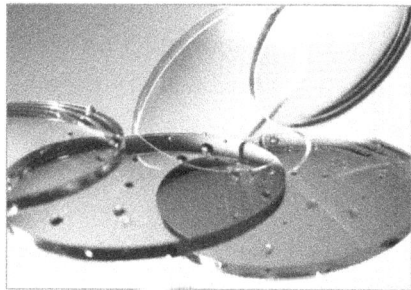

Lens materials

High index is the most common thin lens material. The thinness of high index lenses is characterized by the index of refraction (IR). Mid-high index lenses are commonly around a 1.56IR, high index lenses are around 1.60IR, and ultra-high index lenses are 1.66IR and above. In general, the thinner and lighter the lens, the more expensive it will be.

If the sphere on your prescription is lower than +/-4.00, then hard resin is the best choice for you. If it is above +/-4.00, then high index plastic is best for you. If you are a child or an active adult and need some eye protection, then polycarbonate is best for you. (More about understanding your prescription and what the numbers mean is discussed in depth in a separate chapter. For understanding here, the higher the number, the stronger the prescription, which can often add to the thickness of the lens.)

Polycarbonate lenses are virtually shatterproof and are highly recommended for children and active adults. By active I refer to any activity that includes a possibility of receiving a blow to the face. For example, policemen, firemen, tennis and ball players, and those participating in aggressive sporting activities are at risk—just to name a few. Wearing polycarbonate lenses may not save your eye, but they will certainly help, and a little added protection can't hurt.

In general, if the sphere on your prescription is at +/-2.00 or lower, you will not benefit from the more expensive thin high index lens types. Hard resin or polycarbonate lenses will be just fine for you. If the sphere on your prescription is higher than +/-2.00, you will benefit from the selection of a thin lens type.

Lens thickness chart: Thickness is determined by lens power and lens material.

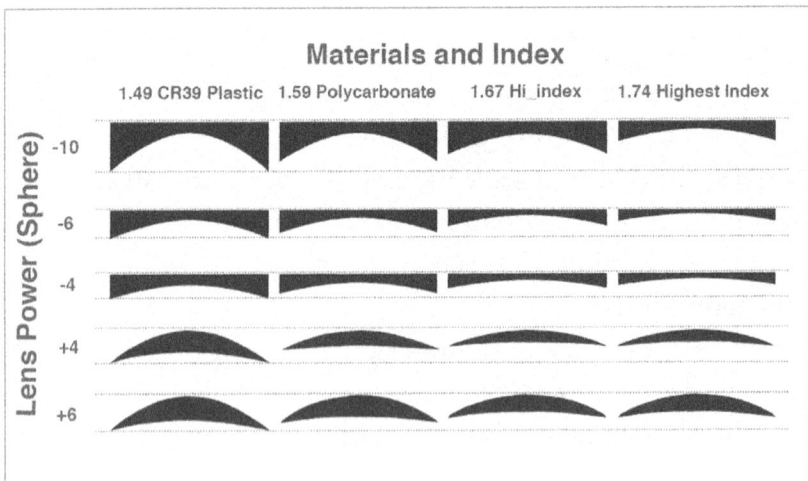

Materials and Index

| | 1.49 CR39 Plastic | 1.59 Polycarbonate | 1.67 Hi_index | 1.74 Highest Index |

Thinner lenses have three advantages: (1) they do not look thick; (2) they do not magnify (make your eyes look larger, and I refer to the Coke bottle taunting many glasses wearers suffered) or minify your eyes (make them look smaller) when seen by others; and (3) they are lighter.

How thick are thin lenses? How thick are the thick ones? The plastic used for lenses in prescription eyewear must have at least a 2.0 mm center thickness according to US law. The thickness at the lens edge depends on the strength of your prescription, your pupil distance, the eye size of the frame, and the lens material.

Because of all of these factors, it is nearly impossible to select a lens by its thinness. There is a lot of advertising around "thin" and "light" lenses, but in actuality, the thinness of a lens is a function of three factors: (1) your prescription, (2) the size and shape of the lens determined by the frame, and (3) the lens material. If your prescription is under +/- 4.00 sphere, there is no reason to pay more for a lens with an index of refraction higher than 1.60. In general, the thinner and lighter the lens, the more expensive it will be, but there are many exceptions to this rule especially if you have a low prescription.

All rimless eyeglasses must use polycarbonate, Trivex (a type of high index lens), or high index lenses to avoid cracking.

After you have selected the best prescription glasses lens material for your personal situation and prescription, you can choose among other lens features and options, like sun-sensitive, scratch coating, anti-reflective coating, and UV protection (UV protection is always inherent in high index and polycarbonate lenses). More on coatings later in this chapter.

If you want sunglasses, additional options could include tint, polarization, and mirror coatings. Additional lens services would include a mounting fee (applies only for rimless frames), and rolling and polishing (applies only to higher power lenses being mounted in certain frame types).

THE MARRIAGE OF FRAME AND LENS

Most frames work with most lenses. There are some exceptions, but only a qualified optical professional can tell you for sure if a lens will work in a specific frame. If your prescription is under +/-4.00 sphere, your lenses will work in almost any pair of frames. If your prescription is stronger than +/-4.00 sphere, or if you want multifocal lenses, there are some additional considerations to make.

Let's look at some basic guidelines (and understand there are many exceptions):

Mild Minus Lenses

If your prescription has a minus sphere (like -4.00, -4.25, or more), hard resin lenses will be noticeably thicker. In this case, you can go to a thinner, more expensive lens material. If you prefer hard resin to save money, you should look for thicker frames in order to cover up some of the edge of the thick lens and avoid thin metal frames that will accentuate thick lenses. Thick lenses are also thicker when wider or taller: you should stick to smaller eye sizes because the bigger the lens size, the thicker it gets at the edge.

Strong Minus Lenses

If you do have a strong minus correction, you should also consider purchasing a thinner lens product, like a high index lens and/ or one with aspheric design. Also, rimless frames are not recommended for thick lenses because the heavy lenses often cause the frames to be top heavy. They'll slide down your nose more readily and can loosen up over time.

Plus Sphere Lenses

If your prescription has a plus sphere (like +4.00, +4.25, or more) you do not need to avoid thin frames since plus sphere lenses are thicker in the middle and thinner at the edge.

Multifocal Lenses

For multifocal lenses (that's progressive, bifocal, and trifocal), there needs to be enough height to the frame (known as the B measurement) so that the viewing areas are large enough to see through. We recommend that the B measurement be at least 30 mm for any frame that will be getting multifocal lenses. If you have fallen in love with frames for glasses with a B measurement of 27 mm to 29 mm, some of the new short corridor lens choices may work for you.

To fit bifocal lenses (and any multifocal lenses) properly, the eyeglasses frames must first be fit and adjusted to your face. At this point, an optical professional measures the segment height of your lenses and makes two dots on the lens, one at the bottom edge of your pupil, and the other at the intersection of the lower cyelid and your eye. The measurement in millimeters from the bottom of the lens up to each dot is the segment height.

To make any multifocal lens, optical technicians must have an accurate segment height measurement. If you send in a pair of glasses with multifocal lenses in them to a lab, techs can read the lens and determine the segment height and make a perfect copy (re-lensing your glasses). But that segment height is specific to each pair of frames and cannot be used for a different pair of frames. You can ask your local optical professional to measure the seg height for a pair of eyeglasses, and then send them to an online store for the lens production.

CHALLENGES AND THE JOY ABOUT PROGRESSIVE LENSES

Progressive lenses were first introduced in the 1990s as a new lens product that offers multifocal vision "without the line." Lens companies realized that aging customers did not like other people seeing the visible bifocal line for cosmetic purposes.

Consequently, the progressive no-line lens was invented and marketed under such names as Varilux, Varilux Comfort, Varilux Definity, Varilux Physio, and many others. This was great news for the eyewear industry because this lens was much more expensive than single-vision or bifocal lenses, which meant more money for the companies selling them.

Optometrists regularly prescribe progressive lenses to people, using their influence with patients as a trusted doctor to prescribe healthy aids. However, progressive lenses do not provide any physiological benefit to patients—only cosmetic benefits—yet they do provide much more money to optometrists. Don't believe me? Have your eyewear professional price out your prescription in both a bifocal and a progressive.

Outside of the cosmetic benefits, progressive lenses offer the convenience of having distance and reading vision in one lens like a bifocal. Unlike a bifocal, however, the progressive lens also offers the midrange and a continuous viewing area in the middle of the lens.

On the negative side, progressive lenses have large areas in the visual field that cannot be seen through, thus causing blind spots, which can lead to headaches and nausea during the adaptation period (it takes time for you to adapt your body and lifestyle to these types of lenses).

Also, to use a progressive lens, you must learn not to move your eyes from side to side, but to move your head from side to side. In most cases, patients are more than capable of learning about eyeglasses and making their own informed choices, along with advice from the eye doctor.

ADAPTING TO PROGRESSIVE LENSES

In order to use a progressive lens, you must learn to move your head to see things; you cannot just move your eyes because you will be looking through a blurry part of the lens. This is called adapting to the lens.

Most people can adapt within a month, but some people never adapt. It is common to experience dizziness and headaches during the time that you are adapting. Getting accustomed to progressive prescription glasses can be difficult, and you must have proper instruction by an eyecare professional.

Sometimes, people who try progressive prescription lenses for the first time have a difficult time learning to look through the appropriate portion of the lens at the right time. Often a simple fitting adjustment to your prescription eyewear by your local optical professional can make all the difference.

COMMON ADAPTATION PROBLEMS
AND SOLUTIONS

It is very common to experience a feeling of disorientation while you adjust to your new glasses, whether they are progressive lenses or not. If you are having trouble adjusting to your new glasses, work through this list in order:

- If your prescription has changed recently, your eyes need extra time to adjust to the new lens.

- If you are wearing multifocal lenses (progressive, bifocal, and trifocal lenses), you must learn to move your head, not your eyes.

- The center of the lenses must be positioned directly in front of your eyes. Make an adjustment to the positioning of the glasses on your face, and be sure the glasses stay in that correct spot.

- If you tried #1 through #3 and you still cannot adjust to your new glasses, it is possible that the pupil distance measurement was taken incorrectly. It is also possible that your eye doctor gave you the wrong prescription (sometimes they do make mistakes!).

- If you tried #1 through #4 and still are not satisfied with your lenses, take the glasses back to the optical store or send them back to the online store so they can double check to be sure that the lenses were made exactly to your specifications.

MORE DECISIONS:
LENS PROTECTION AND COATINGS
Do I need UV Protection?

Ultraviolet (UV) protection and coatings are an important consideration when buying lenses. Most eyeglasses lens materials already have 100% UV protection, and that includes polycarbonate lenses, high index lenses, Trivex lenses, Transitions lenses, and polarized lenses. Lenses that do not have UV protection are the least expensive hard resin CR-39 lenses, and it is important to add a UV coating to these lenses, especially if the glasses will be worn outside.

Most importantly, sunglass lenses that are CR-39 must also have UV protection in the form of UV coating, and this is an

FDA regulation. Cheap flea market sunglasses often do not have UV protection or UV coatings; this is most dangerous because the tint causes the pupils to dilate, and then your eyes admit more UV radiation. Note to self: Don't buy cheap sunglasses.

UV protection and UV coatings in lenses have come to the forefront recently, as Prevent Blindness America has declared May as Ultraviolet Awareness Month to help educate the public on how to protect their eyes from harmful sun rays.

Ultraviolet rays are well known for their damaging effects on the skin, but exposure to UV rays can cause "sunburns" to the eye too—also known as photokeratitis (snow blindness). The damaging effects of UV rays may not develop until years later. In fact, UV damage is cumulative and has been linked to cataracts and macular degeneration later in life. The delicate skin around the eye and the eyelids is also susceptible to UV damage. UV protection and UV coatings in lenses are strongly recommended.

No matter what time of year it is or what the weather forecast is, sunglasses that block 100 percent of UVA and UVB rays should always be worn in conjunction with a brimmed hat. Wraparound sunglasses are best as they protect the eyes and the skin around the eyes. Some contact lenses may offer UV protection, but they can't protect the entire eye and the skin around it.

WHAT IS ANTI-REFLECTIVE (AR) COATING?

Anti-reflective coating (also known as no-glare) is a series of layers that is adhered to the back and front surface of a lens, or just the back of the lens if the lens is polarized. The purpose of no-glare coating is to help reduce the reflections on the lens.

Consisting of metal oxides, each layer is a thin film that is designed to block a specific wavelength of light. The more layers of film, the more wavelengths that are blocked. AR coating causes the light that reflects from the inner and outer surfaces of each film layer to become equal, thereby canceling each other out.

Do you remember back in the 1990s when anti-reflective coatings regularly flaked, stained, and turned psychedelic? It was a nightmare for opticians because customers became angry and would blame them for selling an expensive coating that did not perform well.

Well, the tide has turned and anti-reflective coating is now completely reliable, whether you choose the more expensive Crizal AR coating, or the less expensive AR coatings that are available. Yes, if you leave your glasses on the dashboard of your car in Florida, the anti-reflective coating could show signs of stress, but this falls in the category of abuse.

Anti-reflective coating does cost an additional $20 to $90 depending on the lens it is coating, but there are significant benefits. Whether it is right for you—if it is worth the extra cost—is your decision. Your glasses will work fine without AR coating, but the relaxation to your eyes and improved vision may be worth it.

Crizal is the best known anti-reflective coating on the market, and also the most expensive. Before you choose Crizal (or any number of their specialty coatings), think carefully about whether you even need or want anti-reflective coating on your glasses. Anti-reflective coating is chosen by 28.5% of eyewear shoppers in the United States, compared to 50 to 90% in Europe. My guess is that Americans were turned off by the poor quality of AR coatings three decades ago.

Today's AR coatings include a harder layer of scratch- resistant coating, in addition to oleophobic (anti-oil), hydrophobic (anti-liquid), and anti-static layers. These extra layers help to repel the things that lead to smudging and scratching. They also help to make the lenses easier to clean and thereby reduce surface scratches from excessive cleaning.

Premium AR Coatings

There are basically three types of coatings. Inexpensive coatings are available on a restricted prescription range, because the lenses are coated in a mass production of tens of thousands of lenses. On other lenses that are custom made, there are middle-quality AR coatings, which can offer a one-year anti-scratch warranty. However, it is not quite as good at the premium Crizal AR coatings offered by Essilor.

Anti-reflective coatings always work better when they are made by the same maker as the lens itself. The reason for this is that the manufacturers each have their own formula for the underlying lens. That formula bonds best to an anti-reflective coating that is of the same chemical family. Premium anti-reflective coatings are actually bonded to the lens surface, becoming one with the lens.

Anti-reflective, no-glare coating allows people to see your beautiful eyes

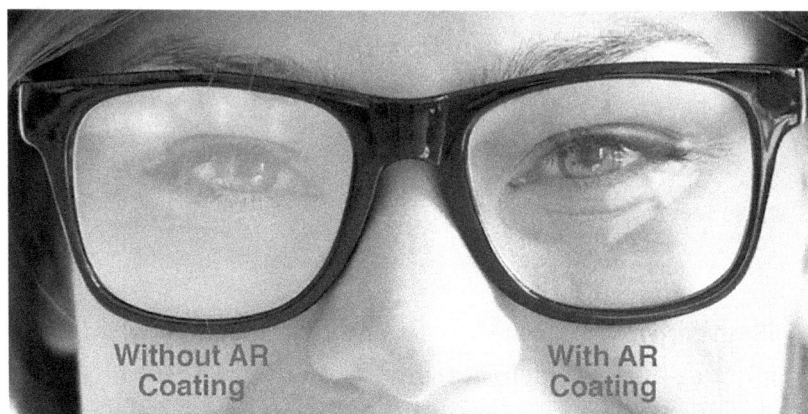

Without AR
Coating

With AR
Coating

Anti-reflective coating allows 8% more light to enter the eye—thus the explanation for the term anti-reflective. And why would you want more light going into your eye, you ask? That 8% of light was bouncing off the outside of the lens, causing other people to see a shiny spot on your glasses and preventing them from seeing your eyes. Also, when a light source is overhead or behind you (as is often the case), light reflects off the inside of your lens and bounces into your eye, increasing eye fatigue.

When there is more available light to your eye, you can see better and more clearly. The result is clearer, sharper vision and reduced eyestrain, which would benefit everyone. However, in some situations, the benefits are more noticeable:

Workplace: Fluorescent lighting, computer screens, and cash registers all cause an increase of reflections in the workplace. This increase in reflections causes eye strain, headaches, fatigue, and a decrease in work productivity. If you work in such a situation, say as a grocery checker, you may want to add AR coating to your glasses.

Anti-reflective, no-glare coating cuts glare in daytime

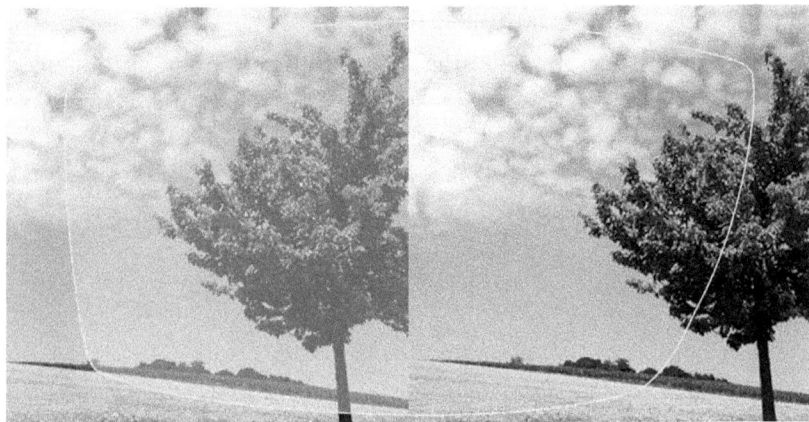

Night driving: External reflections are a major problem when it comes to driving safely at night. The reflections from oncoming headlights, street lights, and the road can cause distractions and discomfort to the driver. Internal reflections can cause ghost images and result in a decrease in reaction time. Consider AR coating for the glasses you wear to drive.

Anti-reflective, no-glare coating cuts glare at night

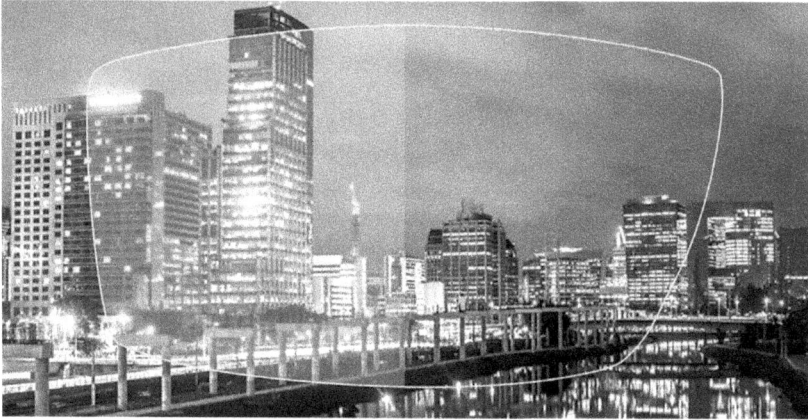

Sunglasses: I highly recommend adding anti-reflective coating on the back side of sunglasses lenses. You see, ambient light is everywhere, and this light gets in behind the glasses and bounces off the lenses and into your eyes. This added glare tires your eyes, causes you to squint more, and also impairs vision. With AR coating on the back side of sunglasses, this light can more easily go through the lens and does not bounce back into your eyes, thus eliminating those problems.

Cosmetic: Without anti-reflective coating, reflections on the lenses will prevent people from seeing your eyes. Actors, newscasters, and business people prefer AR so that their audience and associates can clearly see their eyes.

LENS OPTIONS

Just a few more options to consider before you are good to go with your frames and lens combination. Here are some of the many lens services that are available. Some services are only available on certain lenses and in certain combinations.

Edge polishing: Edge polishing is usually just for rimless frames. Lenses are usually always buffed at the edges, and this service should be included in the basic lens charge. Edge polishing gives a high sheen to the edges of the lens, which some people prefer on the lenses used in rimless frames. In some cases people have lenses that are substantially thicker than the frame and prefer to have a polish on the edges.

Flash mirror coating for sunglasses: Flash mirror coating is a half mirror, so people can still see your eyes. It is fashionable and functional because it cuts glare. The coating is usually available in silver, gold, or blue, but there are also some specialty mirrors available. The flash mirror helps to reduce glare coming off snow, water, and other shiny surfaces. By reducing glare, you reduce eye strain and eye fatigue, which leads to better, long-lasting comfort in glaring circumstances. Flash mirror cannot be applied on top of anti-reflective coating. It is applied on the front of the lens, and the AR coating is applied on the back.

Solid mirror coating for sunglasses: Solid mirror coating is a full mirror. It is fashionable, and it too cuts glare. Coatings are usually available in silver, gold, or blue, but there are also some specialty mirrors available. With full mirror coating, people cannot see your eyes. In fact, people can see themselves perfectly in your mirror lenses and they cannot tell where you are looking. The full mirror helps to reduce glare coming off snow, water, and other shiny surfaces. By reducing glare, you reduce eye strain and eye fatigue, which leads to better, long-lasting comfort in glaring circumstances. Full mirror cannot be applied on top of anti-reflective coating. It is applied on the front of the lens, and the AR coating is applied on the back. If you are in the Secret Service, you probably already have several pairs of glasses with this coating.

Prism: For some people, the eye doctor will add to the prescription something called "prism." If your prescription includes a prism, your lens must be made as a "surfaced" custom-made lens, so there is an additional fee.

Rimless mounting: Rimless, three-piece frames require careful drilling and mounting of lenses. Some frames like the Silhouette rimless frames have a double-drilled hole on each side of each lens. This work is done by hand by skilled technicians who do hundreds of mountings each week. There is usually an additional fee for this service.

Blue-light protection: According to the American Academy of Ophthalmology, the amount of blue light that you would receive indoors is negligible, and there is no proof that it causes eye damage. Additionally, lenses that provide protection from blue light only filter out a small amount of the blue light (10.6% to 23.6%, according to an NIH study).

What is blue light? Excessive blue light (part of the light spectrum closer to UV light) can produce health issues, but moderate amounts of blue light are required for normal body function. In most indoor circumstances, there is no proof that excessive blue light exists, and thus the need to block it has been overemphasized by optical retailers. For more information, visit the website of the American Academy of Ophthalmology (www.aao.org). As new research studies are conducted, the results will be posted on this website.

How Do Photochromic Lenses Work?

Photochromic lenses will darken when exposed to UV light, such as when you walk outdoors. When you are no longer exposed to the effects of UV (let's say you walk indoors), the lenses return to their clear state. Transitions lenses are a brand of lenses made by Essilor, the world's largest lens company, and Transitions photochromic lenses block 100% of harmful UVA and UVB rays. Many people love the convenience of photochromic lenses, as they can have the convenience of both regular eyeglasses and sunglasses in just one pair of glasses.

Photochromic lenses react quickly to changing light and

become sunglasses outside in bright sunlight. As light conditions change, the level of tint adjusts to provide the right tint at the right time. This convenient protection against glare is automatic.

Outdoors, the brighter the sun, the darker the lenses get, all the way to as dark as most sunglasses. So these photochromic lenses help enhance the quality of your vision by reducing the sun's glare in different light conditions—on bright sunny days, on cloudy days, and everything in between. But because extremely high temperatures tend to affect lens performance, some lenses may not always get as dark as sunglasses. Also, since they are activated by UV exposure, some lenses don't work behind the windshield of a car since your windshield actually blocks UV rays.

Because photochromic lenses adjust to changing light conditions and reduce glare, they enhance the ability to discern objects of varying size, brightness, and contrast, enabling you to see better in all light conditions.

Photochromic lenses contain special dyes that cause the lens to activate, or darken, when exposed to ultraviolet rays from sunlight. When the UV light diminishes, the lenses fade back. As light conditions change, the level of tint adjusts, offering the right tint at the right time. It's important to note that the UV radiation blockage remains constant. Photochromic lenses provide automatic protection from UV radiation in both the clear and darkened states.

Most wearers report the adjustment happens so smoothly that they are unaware of it. They are aware, however, of their continued visual comfort.

Photochromic lens products are available for virtually every prescription, material, and lens design. They are also available in shatter-resistant and in standard and high index lens materials. Regardless of your prescription or lens preference, you may choose either gray or brown lenses. Photochromic lenses are also compatible with lens treatments and options such as anti-reflective coating, scratch-resistant coating, and edge polish (which removes the frosted look from lens edges).

FAQS ABOUT FRAMES AND LENSES

Can I buy replacement lenses for my current frames?

Yes, you can replace the lenses in your current frames and save money because you are not buying a whole new frame.

Can I hurt my eyes with the wrong lenses?

There is no clinical evidence to suggest that looking through lenses with the wrong prescription or pupil distance configuration can cause damage to your eyes. However, there could be other undesirable consequences (especially for people with stronger corrections), such as headaches, dizziness, double vision, and vertigo. Some of these effects could cause a dangerous situation if you are driving, handling machinery, or otherwise reliant on your eyeglasses for your safety or the safety of others.

You may experience some of these effects with a new pair of prescription eyeglasses with a stronger prescription you're not used to yet. The effects could fade over time, but I strongly suggest that you visit your local optical professional in order to determine the best course of action.

Can I buy prescription lenses from one store and have them installed elsewhere?

It is highly discouraged. Prescription eyewear lenses cannot be separated from lens installation. Lenses must be purchased and installed by the same company. But let's think about the reverse situation. It is possible to buy prescription frames from one store and have the prescription lenses installed at a different store.

My frames are broken, but my lenses are still good. Can I reuse them?

Prescription glasses lenses can often be re-cut to fit new prescription frames, but there are some restrictions. The new prescription frame must either be the exact same frame model and size as the broken frame, or it must be smaller in every dimension (height and width). Your local optical retailer should be able to examine your prescription lenses and help you select a new prescription frame for them.

Does it matter which lens brand I choose?

Your choice of prescription lens brand is a personal decision, which is generally a trade-off between price and quality. In general, better-quality brand merchandise is more expensive. In prescription lenses, a more expensive lens usually means a better-quality lens, or a lens with a wider viewing area (in the case of progressive lenses). In some cases, however, it may be difficult or impossible for a consumer to notice the difference between a high-quality prescription lens and a low-quality lens. Anti-reflective and scratch-resistance coatings typically adhere better to the lens if they are applied by the lens manufacturer than if applied by a lens laboratory.

How do I order prescription sunglasses?

You can build prescription sunglasses the same way as prescription glasses. Begin by selecting a pair of eyeglasses frames or sunglass frames that can hold a prescription. Lower quality sunglass frames are not designed to hold a prescription lens and are called non-Rx-able. In other words, you can't put a prescription lens in them. Rx-able sunglasses are sunglass frames that can accept a prescription lens. The $19.95 sunglasses you adore and bought on sale at a big box store on a revolving rack are probably not the type you can put a prescription in.

What can I do with glasses I no longer wear?

If you have old eyeglasses that you are not wearing, first check to make sure they are in good working condition and clean. If so, you can donate them to your local Lions Club, which has a nationwide collection system for eyeglasses, which they send to places in the world for people who need them.

4

Magnifying the Problem: Your Close-Up Guide to Great Reading Glasses

Those of us of a certain age find themselves juggling several pairs of readers or "cheaters" in pockets and purses or dangle them around our neck by a cord. Reading glasses is a generic term that refers to glasses that hold lenses used only for reading (near vision).

A reading lens simply magnifies objects that are close to you. Your eye doctor can determine the magnification power that is best for you, or you can figure it out yourself through trial and error. You see those stands of reading glasses at drugstores and discount retailers. Try on glasses with different magnification power until you find a pair (buy two pair, they're cheap) that truly make reading a pleasure again, instead of a struggle. Your arms are just not long enough at some point!

The drugstore readers have the same power in both lenses, right and left. Some people need different powers for each eye, and then you do need to have an optical professional determine your prescription. You can't buy reading glasses, then, off the shelf unless you buy a pair for each power and swap out the lens on one side with the lens from another pair (without breaking the lenses in the process. At $9.99 a pair, your loss would not be too great if you break them).

A doctor's prescription is not required in order to select a reading lens. Drugstore reading glasses are simply glasses frames with lenses preloaded in a range of magnification powers. It is usually less expensive to purchase reading glasses this way, but these stock lens powers may not provide a perfect vision correction for you. (If you have astigmatism, you need prescription reading glasses.)

For best results, reading lenses with magnification customized to your needs can be installed in any pair of glasses frames or prescription sunglasses frames. You can also make your own sun readers for reading at the beach just by asking your optician to add tint to the lenses.

Reading glasses are becoming very fashionable, and many designer frames are now made as reading glasses. Or you can customize a pair of regular prescription designer glasses frames just by adding reading lenses to them.

Reading glasses are finding their way out of the drugstore and into the department store, as more and more people become aware of reading glasses as a fashion accessory. Because you do not need a prescription for reading glasses, you can buy reading glasses online and in many stores. You can buy reading glasses for as little as a few dollars, but the quality of the low-cost reading glasses is quite low.

STOCK VERSUS CUSTOM

The least expensive way to buy reading glasses online is to buy stock reading glasses. These are reading glasses that sit on a rack in many different stores, and you can choose a pair off the rack with your reading power. It is easy to lose reading glasses, so stash them around the home, car, and office and you'll always have a pair around when you need one. Some people prefer folding reading glasses, because folding reading glasses fold up into a small package and are easy to carry.

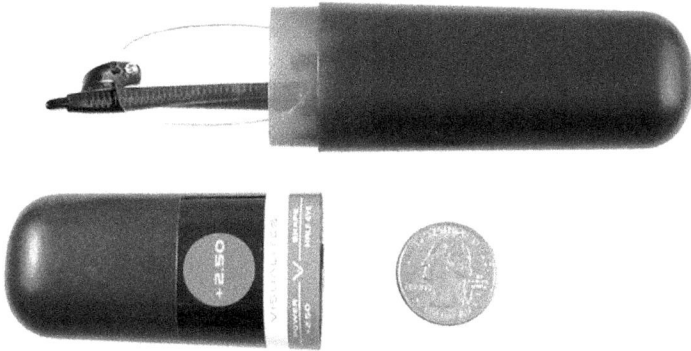

For some people, stock reading eyeglasses may not work well. To get the most effective reading eyeglasses for your eyes, I recommend that you visit an eye doctor to get a prescription for reading. Ask your eye doctor how well served you will be with stock reading eyeglasses, or whether it is better for you to invest in custom reading lenses. Here are some common problems that can occur with off-the-shelf reading eyeglasses:

- Stock reading glasses are made in a one-size-fits-all way. The optical centers of stock reading glasses may be too wide or too narrow for your face. If you don't look through the center of the lens, you may not see clearly and/or you may get headaches or dizziness. I discuss pupil distance as a measurement when fitting frames and lenses elsewhere in this book. If the pupil distance does not work for you, the stock glasses off the shelf at Walmart won't be right.

- Most people do not have the same prescription in each eye, but the lenses of stock reading glasses always have the same power. One side will be fine, maybe, and the other too strong or too weak.

- Many people have astigmatism, which is not corrected in stock reading glasses. This too could lead to not seeing clearly, headaches, and/or nausea.

- Stock reading glasses, especially the $20 variety found in drugstores and superstores, use low-quality plastic lenses that may not be formed properly. The plastic could have blurriness and bubbles, which will impair your vision.

- Reading glasses are designed for a reading focal length of about 12 to 18 inches. Many people buy reading glasses to read the computer screen, which is normally 24 to 36 inches away from your face. Such glasses will make it more difficult for you to see the screen and can cause you to change your posture in your chair, and that can lead to neck strain, back strain, and eye strain. (I have a discussion of computer glasses elsewhere in this book.)

Custom reading glasses are just eyeglasses frames with custom lenses. Typically, this option will be more expensive than buying stock reading glasses, but the quality of the glasses will be much higher and much better suited for your eyes and your lifestyle. To put together custom reading glasses, you need to select a frame and then install lenses.

One thing you cannot do is buy reading glasses at a drugstore and then install custom lenses. The reason is that the frames are not ophthalmic quality. In other words, they are too low quality to accept a custom lens (shall we say cheap?). However, if you have some ophthalmic quality eyeglasses, it is easy to bring them back to life by installing new custom lenses for reading. Why not?

TYPES OF READING GLASSES

Reading glasses are simply magnifying lenses that make objects larger. But there are several different ways to accomplish this goal, so you can choose from a number of different types of reading glasses depending on your lifestyle and needs.

Full-eye and half-eye: With readers, do you want a full frame or a half-eye frame? Full frame reading glasses look like regular eyeglasses, with a frame that goes all the way around the lens, and the lenses sit directly in front of your eyes. Full-eye reading glasses are good when you spend a long time concentrating on material close up. When you look up from reading, objects in the distance appear blurry.

Half-eye: Half-eye reading glasses are flat on the top of the frame and are designed to sit down on your nose so that you look down through the lens when reading. When you look up, you look through air over the lenses, not through a lens, so objects in the distance are not blurry.

Folding readers: Folding reading glasses are designed to take up less space in your pocket or purse. There are many different designs of folding reading glasses. Some—called pen readers or tube readers—are slim and fold into a little tube that you can drop in your pocket. The tube helps to protect the reading glasses from getting crushed.

Rimless: Rimless reading glasses are very practical because your eye does not have to negotiate around the frame around the lens. The edge of the lens obstructs your vision much less than an eyeglasses frame does.

Bifocal readers: Bifocal reading glasses are glasses that have

clear lenses at the top and reading lenses at the bottom. With bifocal reading glasses, you can look straight through the top portion
of the lens without blurriness, and still get reading magnification
when you look down.

Bifocal lenses are available in Standard or Executive designs

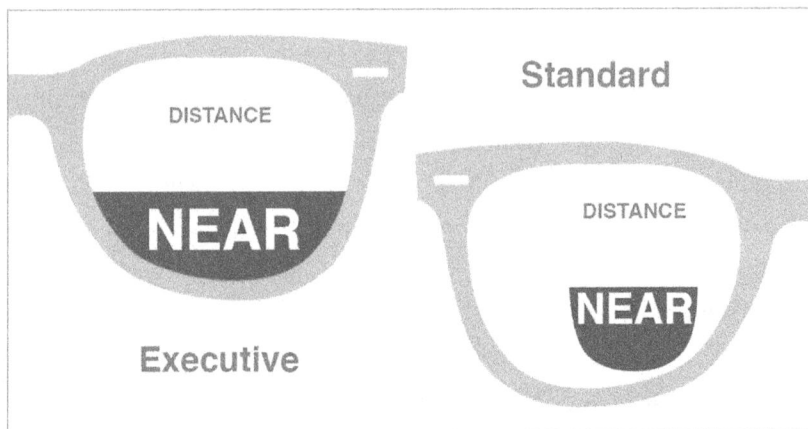

Bifocal no-line readers: Stock reading glasses are available in
a bifocal style, in which there is a line that separates the lower
reading lens from the upper clear lens. No-line reading glasses
perform the same function, but there is no visible line between
the two lens viewing areas. As you move your eyes down from the
upper half, the magnification increases slowly allowing you to see
better at different close-up distances.

Sun readers: Reading glasses with tinted lenses are designed
so that you can read in bright light conditions. For reading in
the sun, many people wear regular sunglasses with contact lenses
underneath. Or you can wear regular sunglasses with stick-on
magnifiers.

Monocles and pince nez: Believe it or not, monocles and pince
nez (pronounced with a French accent as *pants-nay*) are still very
much desired magnification devices. A monocle is a single round

frame that is held in the eye socket (think steampunk Victorian character here, "I say, old chap."). Pince nez means "pinch nose" and the frame literally pinches the side of the nose to hold it in place. Ouch.

5

No More Squinting: Everything You Need to Know about Sunglasses

You can design your own custom prescription sunglasses in the same way that you make your own prescription glasses. Shop for a frame, add a lens with your prescription, and then pick the lens tint and coatings that are best for your needs and lifestyle. Prescription sunglasses are a smart way to see in the sunshine without squinting.

Prescription sunglasses can be made with single-vision, bifocal, or progressive lenses, and in a variety of lens materials and colors. Most prescription sunglasses use the high index polycarbonate lens material, and for high performance prescription sunglasses lenses, I recommend using the Trivex lenses material.

First a word of caution: Lower quality sunglass frames and wrap-style sunglasses are not designed to hold a prescription lens and are called non-RX-able. So RX-able sunglasses are sunglass frames that can accept a prescription lens. Sunglasses frames with an excessive wrap design can only accommodate prescription lenses up to a power of approximately +/-5.00 sphere. You cannot put a prescription in sunglasses with a shield design, which is basically just a single piece of plastic in front of both eyes. Some sunglass manufacturers have facilities to make prescription lenses for their own frames, like Oakley, Bolle, and Maui Jim.

LENS TINTING

Once you have selected a frame, then choose a lens type (hard resin, polycarbonate, high index, polarized, or sun-sensitive). Hard resin and high index lenses can be tinted easily to any color and tint density you choose. You cannot choose the tints for polarized and sun-sensitive lenses; you must choose between brown and gray. Polycarbonate lenses cannot easily be tinted. If you want the durability of polycarbonate lenses in your prescription sunglasses, the lens material to choose is called Trivex. It has the same durability as polycarbonate, but it can be tinted to your desire.

Consider having your optical shop tint the lenses of your old glasses to become sunglasses if you get a new prescription and choose a new frame for your everyday pair.

LENS COLORS

Brown and gray are the most popular colors for sunglass lenses. Brown is the best color overall because it allows the wearer the widest light spectrum through to the eye, while blocking blue light and offering optimum contrast. Brown is suited for applications where distances need to be constantly judged, like tennis or golf or skiing or other sports requiring acute visual perception and contrast differentiation. Brown is also best for lower light situations, like fishing in the late afternoon or early morning.

Gray tint is best for bright light situations like water sports because it blocks out the brightest of the sun's rays.

Other colors like green and blue are used more for fashion purposes than for utility. Blue is the overall worst color of all for the wearer because it enhances blue light, which creates more glare. If you like blue as a fashion choice, consider a custom-made lens tinted brown but with a blue flash mirror coating.

Yellow is used to heighten contrast without blocking too much light, and it is commonly used for shooting and skiing on cloudy days.

Bolle makes a special green tint that is designed specifically for tennis (the Competivision lens) in which the green tint helps to accentuate the yellow color of the tennis balls and make the white lines stand out.

LENS TINT DENSITY

Prescription sunglass lenses are tinted by leaving them in a bath of tint solution. The longer they are left in the solution, the darker the tint becomes. Lenses bathed in tint colors can assume just about any color shade or color density. The lens actually absorbs the tint color into the lens material. Tint density is defined as a percentage, where 0% is completely clear, and 100% permits no light to pass through (solid). A 10% to 20% tint is used for a fashion tint, and a 50% to 80% tint is used for outdoor protection from the sun.

For sun protection, you would use a 50% tint for all-around use, both during midday and during morning and evening hours when there is less available light. For bright light situations, like midday sun on the water, an 80% tint provides maximum protection from the bright sun.

Gradient Tints

A gradient tinted lens has a full tint at the top, fading gradually to no tint at all at the bottom of the lens. A double gradient tint is a lens with a full tint at the top and bottom of the lens, and a medium tint in the center of the lens. Double gradient tints are popular with skiers, because the lens blocks glare coming from above (sun) and below (snow), while allowing for a clearer viewing area in the middle.

Gradient lenses have darker tints at the top, graduating to a lighter tint at the bottom

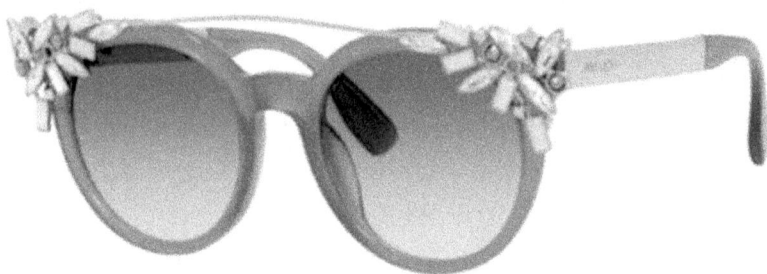

Mirror Coatings

Prescription sunglasses can receive a coating on the outside that looks to others like a mirror. The lens reflects light back and away from the wearer. The advantage of this coating is that it serves to reduce the amount of reflected light or glare that makes it harder to see especially in bright light conditions.

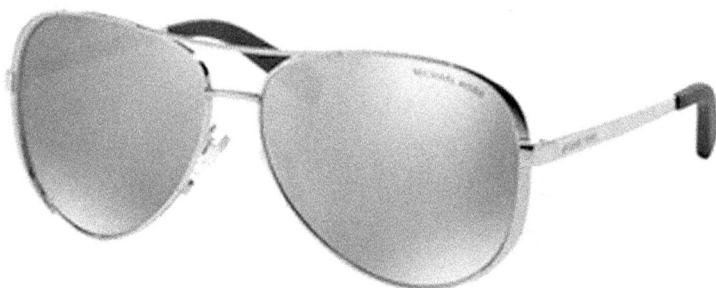

For example, when skiing on a sunny day, there is a lot of reflected light and glare coming off the snow. It is important to

know that the wearer does not see the mirror coating from the inside, but only sees the lens tint. For example, if the lenses had a brown tint with a blue mirror, the wearer would see only brown, and other people would see only the blue mirror. This is a useful combination because, optically speaking, blue is the worst tint for seeing objects clearly (brown is best), but blue is fashionable; so the wearer gets the benefit of seeing through a brown tint as well as the benefit of having other people see only the blue mirror coating.

Mirror coatings are a good alternative to polarized lenses and can be used together with polarized lenses for added protection in extreme conditions. However, using both together will have the effect of darkening the lens and reducing the amount of information your eye receives, which could make it difficult to see in situations where visual acuity is needed (like flying an airplane).

Pure mirror and flash mirror: Mirror coatings are available in two ways, as a flash mirror and as a pure mirror. With a pure mirror, other people will not be able to see your eyes; with a flash mirror lens, other people will be able to see your eyes. The pure mirror is a more intense mirror, and the flash mirror is less intense. In both types of mirrors, the wearer does not see the flash color; the color is only seen by other people.

Polarized Lenses

Polarized lenses are tinted lenses that block vertical light from hitting your eye and causing eye strain. Hunters, boaters and fishermen, golfers, and drivers are the most common users of polarized lenses. Any surface can create glare in sunlight, including water, sand, snow, windows, vehicles, and buildings. Polarized lenses ease eye stress and fatigue in the sun, and lenses are available in several color and density options.

But in some situations, glare can be beneficial. For example, polarized lenses could make it difficult for a driver to see ice on the road, or for a skier to see ice on the ski slope, or for a seaplane pilot to see the water when landing. Polarized lenses function similar to window blinds with horizontal slats when open. You view the slats on the edge so they are very thin, and these edges hold the tint color. Polarized lenses block the vertical light that tries to enter your eye from down below or up above, and it only allows the horizontal light to pass through the lens. Polarized lenses are available in the normal range of vision correction for prescription sunglasses.

SUN-SENSITIVE LENSES

Sun-sensitive lenses are also known by the brand name Transitions, and the technical name photochromic, as discussed earlier. Sun-sensitive lenses automatically darken to a moderate shade when they are exposed to the ultraviolet rays of direct sunlight. When the direct sunlight is removed, the lenses lighten again.

Sun-sensitive lenses are typically only available in brown and gray. Sun-sensitive lenses are available in the normal range of vision correction for prescription sunglasses. A photochromic lens has some limitations you will want to know about.

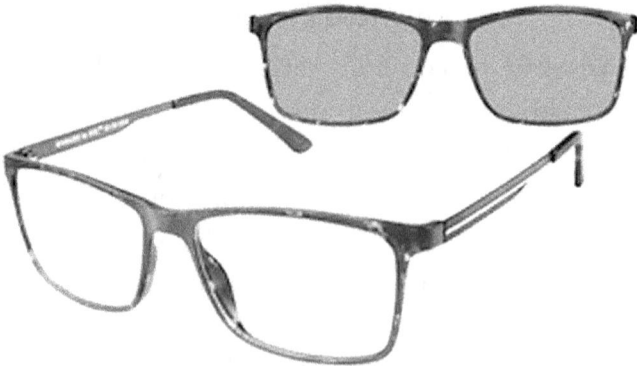

- The lens needs ultraviolet light to darken, and it will darken more slowly or incompletely if the lens is not in direct sunlight. For example, if you are wearing a hat, or if it is cloudy, or if you are inside an automobile, the lenses may darken slowly or not completely.

- It could take up to eight minutes for lenses to transition from dark back to clear. So if you are in and out of the sun, the lenses may not be dark or clear when you want them to be.

- Photochromic lenses do not become completely clear indoors, but retain a light tint that may not appeal to people who want completely clear lenses indoors.

Trivex Sun Lenses

Trivex is a great substitute for polycarbonate lenses in prescription sunglasses, because Trivex can be easily tinted but polycarbonate cannot. Trivex is much better suited for tinting and is an excellent choice for rimless drill-mounted frames. The suggested prescription range is plano (0, no Rx) to +/-8.00 sphere. While Trivex has a slightly lower refractive index than polycarbonate lenses, its specific gravity makes it the lightest of any lens material available today. This means the lens may be a little thicker than polycarbonate lenses but similar in weight. Like polycarbonate lenses, Trivex also has inherent 100% UV protection. However, it is optically superior to polycarbonate lenses, meaning it is much less distortive.

UV PROTECTION

I discussed UV earlier, but it's worth repeating here in reference to sunglasses. Ultraviolet protection and UV coatings are an important consideration when buying eyeglasses lenses. Most lens materials already have 100% UV protection, and that includes polycarbonate lenses, high index lenses, Trivex lenses, Transitions lenses, and polarized lenses. Eyeglasses lenses that do not have UV protection are the least expensive CR-39 lenses, and it is important to add a UV coating to these lenses, especially if the glasses will be worn outside or as sunglasses.

Most importantly, sunglass lenses that are CR-39 must also have UV protection in the form of UV coating, and this is an FDA regulation. Cheap flea market sunglasses often do not have UV protection or UV coatings; this is most dangerous because the tint causes the pupils to dilate, and then your eyes admit more UV radiation. Note to self: Don't buy cheap sunglasses.

UV protection and UV coatings in eyeglasses lenses have come to the forefront recently, as Prevent Blindness America has declared May as Ultraviolet Awareness Month to help educate the public on how to protect their eyes from harmful sun rays. Think of it as sunscreen for your eyes.

Ultraviolet rays are well known for their damaging effects on the skin, but exposure to UV rays can cause "sunburns" to the eye too—also known as photokeratitis (snow blindness). The damaging effects of UV rays may not develop until years later. In fact, UV damage is cumulative and has been linked to cataracts and macular degeneration later in life. The delicate skin around the eye and the eyelids is also susceptible to UV damage. UV protection and UV coatings in lenses are strongly recommended.

No matter what time of year it is or what the weather forecast is, sunglasses that block 100 percent of UVA and UVB rays should always be worn in conjunction with a brimmed hat. Wraparound sunglasses are best as they protect the eyes and the skin around the eyes. Some contact lenses may offer UV protection, but they can't protect the entire eye and the skin around it.

ANTI-REFLECTIVE (AR) COATING

AR coating goes on the backside (side closest to your face) of prescription sunglasses and nonprescription sunglasses. Backside AR prevents light and glare from coming in to either side and from behind you, bouncing off the inside of the lens and into your eye. This kind of glare is very common in sunny situations. Add this type of coating to eliminate this glare from your vision.

CLIP-ON SUNGLASSES

Clip-on sunglass lenses are tinted lenses that clip on to regular prescription glasses, effectively turning them into prescription sunglasses. The clip-ons usually match the eyeglasses frame in shape and color and attach either by clips or with magnets. Regular clip-ons require two hands to add and remove the clips, but magnetic clip-ons (they hold to the frame with magnets instead of clips) can be added or removed with just one hand. Other clip-ons may just flip up and remain attached.

Clip-ons have advantages and disadvantages. It is convenient to be able to convert your eyeglasses into sunglasses and back again. However, wearing a clip-on means adding a significant amount of reflected glare. Light passes through the clip, reflects off the front of the frame, reflects off the back of the clip, and bounces around in there, causing significant additional glare and eyestrain that does not occur with prescription sunglasses.

You've seen the sunglasses that are designed to fit over your eyeglasses, covering them completely. Fit-overs are useful for eyeglasses that do not have matching clip-ons, and they also serve to block out light from entering around the sides of your glasses. Side-glare is extremely annoying, especially on the water, so fit-overs may be a better solution for sun protection than clip-ons.

6

Understanding Specialty Glasses

KIDS AND GLASSES

The most important issues in choosing glasses specifically for children are safety, durability, cost, and wear. Regarding safety, children should only wear polycarbonate lenses. Cost and durability are related; you should not pay a lot for children's glasses because kids are likely to damage or lose them, and they will certainly outgrow glasses just like they outgrow shoes.

To limit these problems, look for spring hinges that allow for some flexibility and help to avoid breakage at the temples. Stronger frame materials like titanium or flexible frames will last longer, but generally cost more. You may want to buy two pairs of cheaper frames for glasses and lenses instead of one pair of expensive frames.

If your child is very active, you should consider cable temples that hold the frames for glasses to the ears better, but these can also be annoying and painful behind the ears. Finally (and most importantly) your child is more likely to wear the frames for glasses if he or she likes them.

Online Glasses Shopping for Children

Shopping for frames online for children is more difficult (but not impossible) because of the special considerations for smaller children. The most important place to start is with the current frames they are using. Find out the size of the glasses (I explained where to find these numbers earlier), and then use the advanced search tool on websites to find frames with a similar or somewhat larger size.

To make eyeglasses, an accurate pupil distance measurement is required every year for a child, and sometimes every six months until the child stops growing.

BETTER BE SAFE WITH SAFETY GLASSES

Safety glasses are designed to protect your eyes from certain hazardous tasks. If you are looking for safety glasses, the first thing you need to define is what you are trying to protect your eyes from. This is essential to determine the right piece of equipment to use for your eyes.

There are two parts to safety glasses: the frame and the lens. Your purpose for the glasses will determine what type of frame and what type of lens will solve your problem. For example, if you are using a chainsaw, you will need a strong frame and strong lenses. A safety frame will not break upon impact and is made of material different from a regular frame.

In lenses, again, your goals should determine the type of lens you need. If you are working around chemicals, then you will need a lens that can stand up to such chemicals. This may require a glass lens or a specialty lens.

Most lenses for safety glasses are made out of polycarbonate, which is a standard lens material. It can stand up to most applications, like cycling, sports, and construction applications.

The main consideration when purchasing safety glasses is comfort and coverage. Comfort includes how it feels on your face. Ask yourself: Do these glasses fit well? Are they light? Is there good air circulation so the glasses do not fog up when I sweat?

Coverage means that the lens should cover your eyes completely. This means a close fit at the forehead, cheeks, and sides. If your safety glasses do not provide good coverage, then they are not doing their job of protecting your eyes.

For people who also need vision correction, finding safety glasses with prescription lenses becomes much trickier. Frames with lenses that provide good coverage often are not available with prescription lenses. In order to cover the sides of your face, the lens needs to "wrap" around the side, and it is not possible to make prescription lenses *for wrap-style frames.*

You have two options to solve this problem: (1) Find a safety frame with an optical clip-in insert. The prescription is installed in the clip, which then clips inside the larger safety lens that wraps around your face, or (2) use a goggle-type frame that covers your eyes completely but eliminates your peripheral vision and has a prescription lens in the front. Many motorcyclists use this type. The problem with the goggle style is that it does tend to get hot so it does not work well in sporting applications.

How to Buy Safety Glasses

If you have a specialty application for your safety needs (at-home construction projects, for example), you should definitely start by having a personal discussion with an optical professional. If you are looking for a more generic application—let's say for cycling or sports—there are many options available, and the best method is simply trial and error to find the combination of features that protects your eyes and frames that fit comfortably and are also fashionable.

7

Best Ways to Fit and Take Care of Your Glasses

LET'S TALK ABOUT FIT

Fitting eyeglasses frames begins with this question: "Do you like the way the glasses look on your face?" If you like the way the glasses look on your face, and the frames are comfortable, then you don't need to do anything else.

If the eyeglasses frames are not comfortable or are slightly crooked, an optical professional can make minor adjustments to the bridge, nose pads, and temples to customize the eyewear to the uniqueness of your face. If you have a stronger prescription, I recommend that you have your eyeglasses fitted by an eyecare professional.

Eyeglasses frames often need to be adjusted to your face in order to stay in the correct place and be as comfortable as possible. All eyeglasses frames are designed with materials that can be adjusted. Temples, temple corners, nose bridge, and nose pads are all designed for adjustment. Eyeglasses and sunglasses are designed to be adjusted (bent), if necessary, to accommodate most any facial structure. When a local optical professional is adjusting your eyeglasses for you, it is called a fitting.

How Opticians Adjust and Fit Eyewear

I recommend that you visit a qualified eyecare professional to have your frames fitted properly. This is the best practice but is not a requirement. Many opticians will fit your frames free of charge, or they may charge a nominal fee if you didn't buy the glasses from them. A proper fitting by an eyecare professional is important to ensuring the comfort of your eyewear. An optician begins by aligning and "truing" eyeglasses frames, so that they are even from every angle, with the frame front slightly curved (face form) and the bottom of the frame closer to the face than the top (pantoscopic tilt).

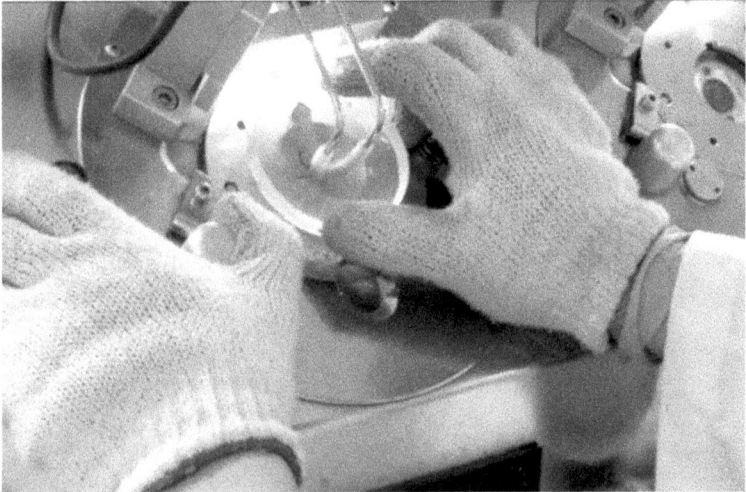

Brand new glasses are almost always aligned and trued at the factory. In the rare case in which new frames are out of alignment, the optician bends the frame into proper alignment using a combination of hands, pliers, and heating equipment (for plastic frames). The next step in the fitting process involves adjusting a "true" pair of frames for the unique characteristics of your face. Eyeglasses fit properly when they feel comfortable to the wearer, and the lenses are equidistant from the face.

Once this position has been established, the optician checks to be certain the lenses are positioned in the correct spot in front of your pupil. The characteristics of your prescription determine the special details that need to be adjusted by a qualified eyecare specialist.

Fitting for Progressive, Multifocal, or Bifocal Lenses

Multifocal lenses (progressive, bifocal, or trifocal) all have a line that divides the distance vision lens from the near vision lens. The line may be visible in the case of a bifocal, or invisible in the case of a progressive lens.

The optician must determine the correct position for this line, by marking on the demo lenses the segment or seg height—the height from the bottom of the lens up to the correct position for the line. In order to determine the correct seg height, the optician must fit and adjust the frames on the wearer's face. The seg height will be different for every pair of glasses and can only be determined after the eyeglasses have been fit to your face by an optical professional. As a result, the seg height must be measured again for every pair of glasses.

HOW TO ADJUST GLASSES YOURSELF

If you do decide to adjust your eyeglasses yourself, I caution that you must be extremely careful. The adjustable parts of eyeglasses are small and thin. If your adjustments are done in the wrong way, you can damage the eyeglasses, void the warranty, and the manufacturer or retailer will not replace them. If you adjust your eyeglasses too often, the metal may fatigue and break.

Why Do You Need to Adjust Glasses?

If you have bought eyeglasses online, before you begin your eyeglasses adjustment, be sure you know exactly what it is you want to accomplish. The two most common goals are to position the optical center of the lens directly in front of your pupils, and to make wearing the glasses feel more comfortable on your face.

To get the optical center of the lenses directly in front of your eyes, first stand in front of a mirror and look straight ahead, neither up nor down. Put on your eyeglasses and position the center of the lenses directly in front of your eyes. Be sure to look straight ahead when you do this. This shows you the place on your nose that you want the frames on your face. Now, you need to adjust your frame so that it will always be correctly positioned.

My frame has nose pads, now what? You can adjust the nose pads so that they keep the frame in the right place. Widening the nose pads drops the glasses lower down on your nose. Bringing the nose pads closer together raises the glasses up on your nose. Nose pads are attached to nose pad arms, which are welded to the frame. You should make only tiny adjustments to the nose pad arms. If you make large adjustments, or frequent adjustments, the arms will break or the weld to the glasses frame will break.

If your frame does not have nose pads, you only need to adjust the temple tips in order to accomplish your goal. Frames without nose pads can be more difficult to position in the correct place, because they lack the adjustability of the nose pads.

On metal or plastic eyeglasses, adjustments to the temples should be small and infrequent in order to avoid fatiguing the frame. Opticians use special equipment to warm up the temples, along with special tools, to make the bend in the exact correct place without fatiguing or breaking the parts.

CLEANING GLASSES THE RIGHT WAY

Grandma used a little spit or breath and the corner of her apron to clean her glasses. Of course, that's not the best way to clean them. Cleaning eyeglasses properly takes time and patience. The sure way to scratch your eyeglasses frames or lenses is with improper cleaning. For example, the people who have chronically scratched lenses are the ones who clean their lenses in the worst possible ways.

Cleaning eyeglasses frames is best done with warm soapy water. If you clean just the lenses, the dirt and facial oils from the frame will eventually find their way to the lenses. You can also take your prescription glasses to a local optical store, which has a machine for cleaning frames. However, if your frame has any inlaid gems, you should not have them cleaned by machine, only by hand.

Here is the smart way to clean your glasses:

1. Warm soapy water. Hold the frames under a faucet of warm water. Get your fingers soapy and gently rub the lenses and the frame. This will remove grease and dirt without scratching the lenses.

2. Lens cleaner. You can use lens cleaner from a small spray bottle if it is more convenient, but we at Eyeglasses.com prefer the water method if at all possible.

3. Gently dab dry. The biggest mistake people make is to rub too hard. Rubbing hard, especially on a dry lens, is where most of the scratches come from. Gently dab the cloth on the lens until it is dry.

4. Use a soft cloth. The best cloth to use is a microfiber cloth. If that's not available, use a clean cotton cloth. And if that's not handy, you

can use a tissue or toilet paper, even paper towels, followed by sandpaper (just kidding). If your cloth is not soft, the lenses will scratch. If your cloth is not clean, the lenses will scratch.

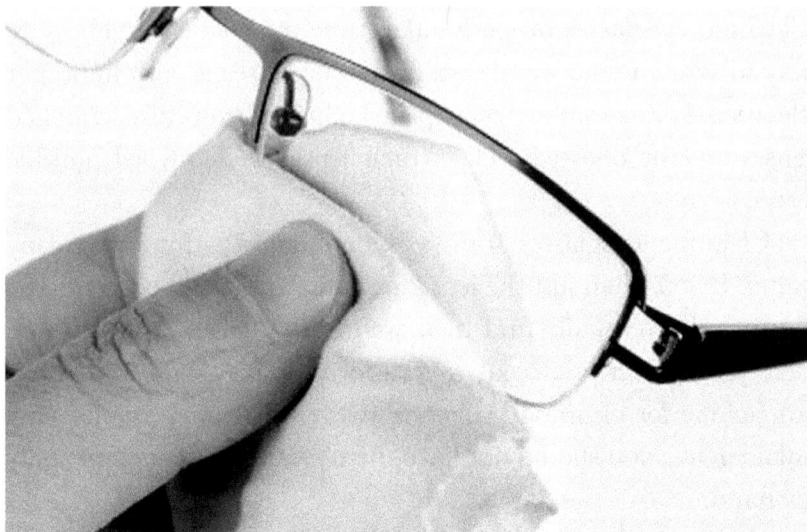

REPLACING BROKEN GLASSES

Even though your eyeglasses frame is broken, you can still save those expensive lenses by putting them into a new frame. Some optical stores offer a personal service to find a new frame that will fit your lenses, but many stores will try to force you to buy a whole new set of lenses.

Eyeglasses lenses are specifically made for your face and the original frame you chose. If the frame breaks, it may be possible to find another frame that will fit the lenses, but it requires extra work. Your first step is to try to find the exact same frame. Going to the internet is the best place to start. Search for the brand name and model name/number. If you can find the frame on the internet, buy it, because the chances are remote that your local optical will have that exact frame.

If that is not possible, find a friendly optical store or online customer service person to help you. Frames that are similar to yours may work, but there are several considerations and only a qualified optician will be able to find a workable replacement. If a replacement can be found, you will save a considerable amount of money by not having to start over with your lenses.

It is important to note here that this is a good reason not to purchase low-quality, cheap eyeglasses in the first place. What happens if you install expensive lenses into a frame that breaks due to cheaply made hinges, nose pads, screws, or some other part?

Of course, if lenses are scratched beyond repair, you can use the frames again and buy replacement lenses.

EYEGLASSES CASES

When you buy a new pair of eyeglasses, an eyeglasses case should be included free of charge. All designer brands of eyeglasses provide cases designed to fit your eyeglasses. The provided case could be hard shell, soft shell, fabric, cloth, or a combination of these. Lower quality frames typically do not have a case to go with them; the dispensing optician may provide a generic case or may try to charge you extra for it.

A hard case is useful to protect your glasses if you are going to carry them in a place where they could get scratched or crushed. However, a hard case does have some disadvantages: (1) It is larger and takes up more space; (2) it can be harder to open if you have trouble with your fingers; or (3) sometimes a hard case with a strong closure can snap shut and injure your fingers.

Soft cases are smaller, making them more suited for a purse because they take up less space. However, many soft cases have some kind of button or other closure that must be closed and opened when you use your glasses. Annoying.

Cloth cases are the smallest option and do a good job of protecting frames and lenses from small scratches, but cloth cases won't provide any protection from crushing. Some cloth cases can also be used to gently clean eyeglasses lenses because they are made from microfiber cloth designed for that purpose.

Who's Who in the Optical Industry

Buying eyeglasses always begins with a prescription. Just as a medical doctor can write a prescription for medicine, the eye doctor can write a prescription for your vision correction. This is a regulated and monitored industry. Not just anybody can judge which correction you need to see better. A prescription can be issued by an optometrist (OD) or ophthalmologist (MD), and you can buy glasses from them, or from an optician, optical professional, or anywhere else.

EYE DOCTORS AND OTHERS

Who is an ophthalmologist (MD)? An ophthalmologist is a medical doctor who has spent four years of medical school followed by at least three years of residency, just like your family practice physician. They are qualified to perform eye surgeries, diagnose and treat eye diseases, dispense all kinds of eye-related medications, write prescriptions for eyeglasses and contact lenses, and do everything that is eye-related.

However, in reality, like most professionals, ophthalmologists are good at some things, and not so good at others. Due to their education and experience, ophthalmologists prefer and excel at eye-related medical work. They are not as skilled at producing really good prescriptions or at dispensing eyewear. Prescriptions issued by ophthalmologists need to be changed more often than prescriptions issued by optometrists.

If you have eye diseases such as cataracts or glaucoma, you need to be seeing an ophthalmologist.

Who is an optometrist (OD)? An optometrist has completed four years of optometry school and the DO stands for Doctor of Optometry (look for their diploma; most display them on the wall in their clinics). They are not qualified to perform surgeries, but can do many diagnostic tests. They can dispense certain medications, eyeglasses, and contact lenses, and of course issue prescriptions. About 90% of optometrists also dispense eyewear. Optometrists are often referred to as "doctor." And this is the person generally referred to as an eye doctor.

Who is an optician? About twenty-five states in the United States do not have laws requiring opticians to be licensed. And

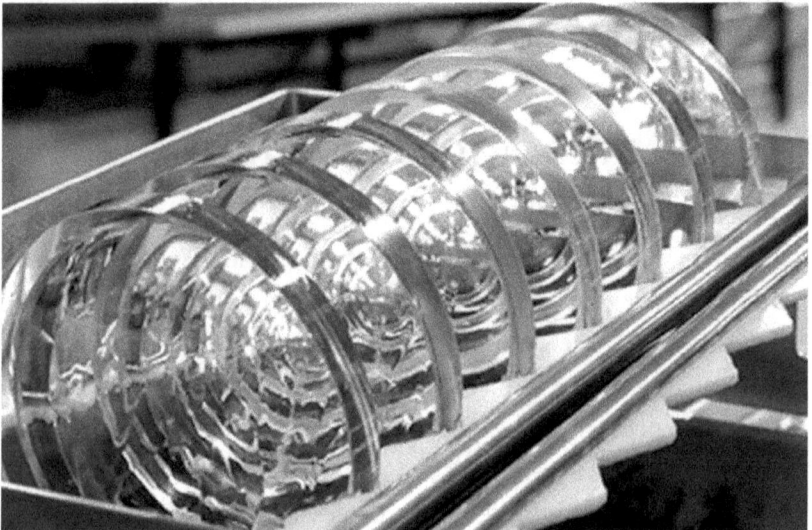

some of the states that do require a license do not require vigorous training. Other states, like Connecticut, have rigorous requirements, like two full years of school followed by a very difficult examination in both eyeglasses and contact lens dispensing. This has led to a great disparity in eyeglasses pricing (higher in the licensed states) and eyeglasses dispensing quality (lower in the unlicensed states).

A licensed optician (LO) has received a license from a state. In some states like Connecticut, those requirements are intense. In other states, like New Hampshire, there are no technical skills, training, or examination requirements. A certified optician is a designation that is available usually in a state without licensure or training requirements, but indicates that a person has received an additional level of training and education.

Licensed opticians, certified opticians, opticians, and optical professionals cannot write prescriptions or dispense medications. They can only dispense eyewear and fit glasses and, in some places, contact lenses.

In some optical offices, you may see an optometrist for your eye exam and then an optician to help you choose eyeglasses. Or you may see the optometrist for your eye exam and prescription and then shop around, including online stores, for your frames and lenses.

Who are the laboratory technicians that make the lenses? Somebody, somewhere actually makes the lenses that fit into the frames you have chosen. Making perfect eyeglasses is a science and an art rolled into one.

Eyeglasses lenses are nothing more than a carefully carved block of clear plastic. Lens quality is determined by four factors: the clarity of the plastic, the precision of the carving, the accuracy of the prescription and PD measurement, and the accuracy of the cutting of the lens to fit your frames.

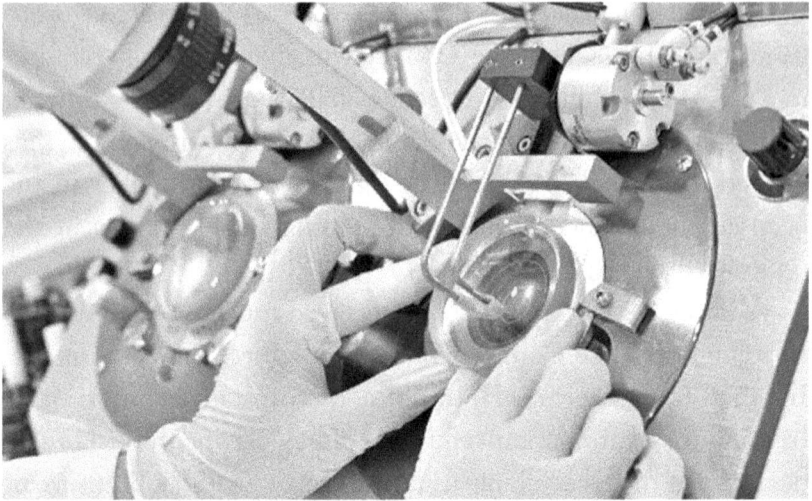

Several groups are involved in the making of lenses. A problem in any one of these steps can lead to less effective vision correction by the lens. A good provider of eyeglasses lenses will have relationships with the best lens quality providers but will also check and re-check every lens before dispensing it. The store you choose to make your lenses must insist on quality at every level in order for you to receive the best quality product. This kind of quality control is essential in order to ensure consistent results.

The maker of the plastic determines the clarity of the plastic. The cutter of the plastic determines the precision of the carving. The plastic maker does the surfacing for stock lenses. The lens laboratory does the carving for surfaced lenses.

The eye doctor determines the optics for the lens such that it will work best for your eyes. An eyewear store employee measures the pupillary distance.

The person who cuts ("edges") the lens for your frame installs lenses so that the optical centers match the pupillary distance measurement. This could be an eyewear store employee or lens laboratory.

Edging is performed in a number of different ways. It can be done at the lens laboratory, or in the optical store. Either way, it is not required in any state that the edging be done by a licensed person. About half of the states in the United States have opticianry laws. In those licensed states, edging can be done by an unlicensed person who is "overseen" by a licensed person. The edging for most glasses made in this country is not performed by a licensed professional.

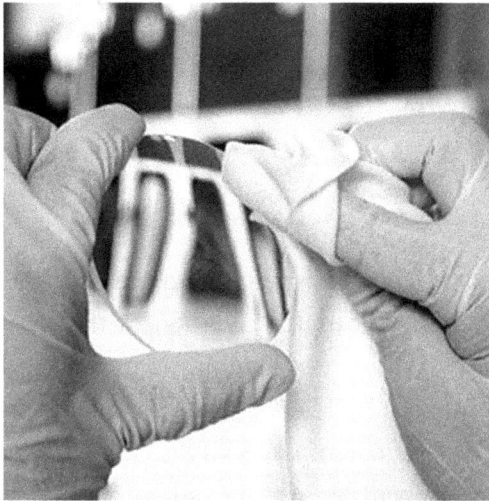

Most quality lens plastic is made in the Far East. It is made in large pieces called blanks, which are round and about four inches in diameter and about half an inch thick. There are different types and qualities of blanks. The quality is determined by the clarity, meaning the absence of miasms (small bubbles or inconsistencies that can only be seen with a microscope). The lower lens quality and less expensive plastics have more miasms, which, although you cannot see them with the naked eye, can still add up to decreased visual acuity. It is very easy for any eyewear retailer to cut their lens costs by 90% by switching to lower quality lens suppliers.

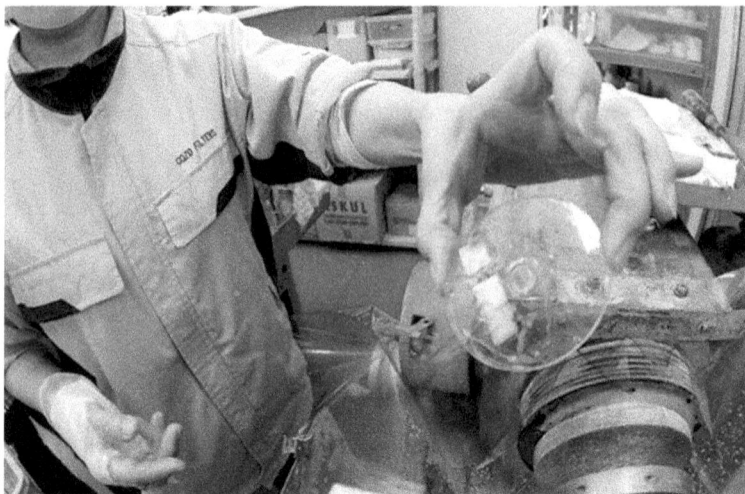

There are two basic ways of cutting lenses, depending on the prescription. Most prescriptions fall within a standard range, called the stock range (on average the range is +/-8.00 sphere and up to +2.00 cylinder). Single-vision lenses that are in the stock range are usually surfaced by the plastic makers in bulk by huge computerized machines. These lenses are then shipped to optical stores so that the store employees can edge the lenses into the frame. Most multifocal lenses, and all lenses that fall outside of the stock prescription range, must be fashioned custom for each prescription. In these cases, plastic blanks (chunks of plastic) are shipped to lens laboratories where they are carved (surfaced) for each individual prescription.

There are hundreds of lens laboratories around the country, several in each state. A typical lens laboratory will do a minimum of a few hundred lenses a day with a large staff of highly trained and experienced technicians. A few optical stores (like LensCrafters) have small surfacing facilities in each of their stores doing much smaller lens volume. To surface a lens, the lens laboratory takes the blank and puts it through a series of grinding machines, which grinds the surface of the lens and shapes it exactly to the specifications of the prescription.

Lens laboratories also provide other services like edging and mounting, which optical stores can choose to use or not, depending on whether they want to do that work themselves. As with any custom service, the quality of the surfacing and any other services that the lab provides is determined by the experience and the expertise of the laboratory, its personnel, and the equipment it uses. If you ask your optical store, you want to hear that they use a lab that employs a large staff of highly trained technicians, doing a large volume of lenses every day.

HOW TO READ AND UNDERSTAND YOUR EYEGLASSES PRESCRIPTION

Prescriptions have a certain format that is always followed. The first line of your prescription is always for the right eye,

Prescription forms vary, but the information is always in the same format

GLASSES PRESCRIPTION

Patient

Expiration Date

		SPHERE	CYLINDER	AXIS	PRISM	BASE	ADD
DISTANCE	OD						
	OS						

ADDITIONAL INFORMATION

Prescribed by _____

sometimes designated the OD. The second line is for the left eye, sometimes designated OS. The prescription for each eye is divided into sphere, cylinder, and axis values. It is common to have no values for any one of these, in which case you might see the letters PL or Plano, or to have values for all of these. Sometimes the prescription may say OU, which means both eyes.

Multifocal Prescription

If your prescription is for bifocals or trifocals or progressive lenses, there may be additional information on the prescription that says for example add +2.50. This is important information if you are ordering reading or multifocal lenses. The numbers are expressed in diopters that tells the power of the lens. A diopter is a value that is metric and universal worldwide.

On a prescription for multifocal lenses, for example, you will see information designated as add power. Your add power is simply the magnification that is added to your sphere value for distance vision, in order to create a field of view for reading. For example, if your sphere value for distance viewing is 3.00, and your add power is +2.00, then your near vision correction is 1.00. Or if your sphere value for distance viewing is +1.00 and your add power is +2.00, then your near vision correction is +3.00.

Don't worry if you don't understand the numbers and their values, but understand this: The optometrist or ophthalmologist that issues the prescription is not involved in the fashioning of the lens, but the prescription they issue is crucial to the overall effectiveness of the lens. Occasionally the OD or MD can issue a prescription that is not quite right. Also, it is possible for your eyes, and your prescription, to change rapidly during some stages of your life. If you just don't think your correction is working in your new glasses, see the issuer of the prescription for a further check.

When an eye doctor provides you with your prescription, that information belongs to you and you should leave the doctor's office with a copy of your glasses prescription. The glasses prescription can be used on any kind of eyeglasses; your glasses prescription is not restricted to glasses that may be recommended by the doctor or sold to you in the doctor's optical shop.

The Missing Number You Need to Know: Pupil Distance, PD

Your prescription should include a pupil distance measurement (also called pupillary distance and shortened to PD). Some offices will try to prevent customers from getting access to their pupil distance measurement in order to make the eyeglasses sales, but this practice is deceptive and illegal. If you have your eyeglasses prescription with your pupil distance noted when you leave your eye doctor's office, then you can buy glasses with that prescription at any eyewear store anywhere.

Normally an optical store employee will take your PD measurement when you buy glasses. If you want more freedom to choose where to buy your eyeglasses, you should ask your optometrist or ophthalmologist to measure the PD during your exam. Usually they will not measure the PD unless you ask them to. With your PD and your prescription, you will not be forced to go to an optical store to get your PD measurement, and then feel obligated to buy glasses from that store.

An accurate pupil distance is a required measurement in order to make prescription glasses, and you cannot purchase eyeglasses without one. Your PD is the distance in millimeters between your pupils (the centers of your eyes), and this number varies from person to person. Your adult PD never changes, and it averages 60 millimeters (mm) for women, and 64 mm for men. Sometimes your eye doctor will write your PD for each eye (for example 33/34, called a monocular PD). Or the eye doctor may write the

PD as 67/64. This means that your PD for distance vision (or DPD) is 67, and for near vision (or NPD, for reading eyeglasses or multifocal lenses) is 64. Your near vision PD is almost always 3 mm less than your distance vision PD.

How is PD measured? The pupil distance is measured with a box-like instrument called a pupillometer (of course) that is put up to your face. Any optical store employee can measure your pupil distance with this instrument. It is not a measurement that is required to be taken by an eye doctor. Any optical store will have a pupillometer, so eye doctors assume that you will have your pupillary distance measurement taken in the optical store. Write that number down on your prescription.

How to measure your own PD using the ruler method. You can follow these easy instructions and measure your own PD with the help of a friend. However, I strongly recommend that you have an eyecare professional measure your pupil distance with a pupillometer. For strong prescriptions, this is a requirement. For weak prescriptions, here are some instructions for measuring your own pupillary distance.

Ask your friend to do the following:

- Find a ruler with millimeter measurements and hold it up to the bridge of your nose.

- Have your friend close one eye.

- Your friend should align the ruler's zero on the left, in the center of your pupil. The pupil is the black spot in the middle of your eye.

- Without moving the ruler, have the friend move their head to the right and read the millimeter line corresponding to your other pupil.

- Repeat the process two or three times for accuracy.

- Record your results.

How to measure your own PD using the photo method. The photo method also works, but like the ruler method, it is not as accurate as having an optical professional measure it with an instrument.

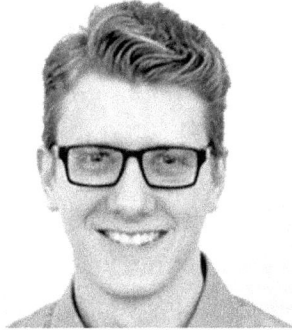

Put on your glasses and take a picture

Step 1: Find a pair of eyeglass frames that have the size number printed on them. Put them on and take a picture of your eyes, as big a picture as you can make.

Step 2: Read the size numbers from the frame, and write down the eye size and bridge size. It should look something like this on the frame: 50 15 145. The first number is the eye size (width of one lens in millimeters) and we will call this the "E" value.

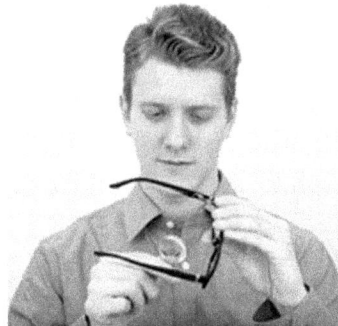

Read the eye size from the numbers printed on your frame

Step 3: Hold a millimeter ruler up to your picture. Measure the width of one lens (do not include the frame, just use the

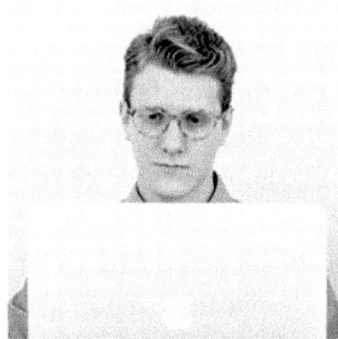

Use a ruler to measure the millimeters of a lens in your picture, and then the millimeters from one pupil to the other

lens width at its widest point). We will call this the "L" value.

Step 4: Hold the ruler up to the picture and measure the distance between your pupils (the black dots in the middle of your eyes). If your pupils are large, measure from the center of each pupil. We will call this the "P" value.

Step 5: Make the formula: $PD = P \times E/L$.

How to measure your own PD using the online method. Some websites now use facial recognition to determine the PD. Basically, you take a picture holding a credit card in front of your face, and the application automatically finds your eyes and measures your PD. Several applications can do this, and you can find them by inputting this search query into a search engine: "pupil distance measurement app." As with the other methods, accuracy is important when making lenses, especially if your prescription has a sphere and/or cylinder value over +/- 2.00.

CLEAR VISION ABOUT THE EYE TESTS YOU NEED—AND WHEN

Across cultures and national boundaries, sight is valued as the most important of the five senses. But new research reveals that across the world, nearly half of adults share the misguided belief that seeing well translates to good eye health. This and other findings confirm a large global gap between vision care attitudes and behavior, which may be preventing people from seeking proper treatment and diagnosis for them and their children.

Despite these reported beliefs, however, only half of survey participants have ever had a comprehensive eye exam—an examination conducted in an office by an eyecare professional that checks not just for vision correction needs, but also for overall eye health.

More than 1 in 3 parents/caregivers have never taken their child under eighteen years of age for any type of vision assessment.

Regardless of your age or your physical health, a routine eye test is important for general health maintenance—even if you don't think you need vision correction with glasses. In addition to evaluating a person's eyes for glasses and contacts for the right prescription, during an eye exam the optometrists or ophthalmologists will check your eyes for eye diseases and other problems that could lead to vision loss.

A wide variety of vision tests and procedures are used to examine the eyes ranging from simple assessments such as having the patient read an eye chart, to complex tests such as a corneal and retinal topography vision test for conditions such as astigmatism, or an eye test to evaluate the blood circulation in the retina. In addition, eye doctors frequently are the first healthcare professionals to detect chronic systemic diseases such as high blood pressure and diabetes, which can seriously affect a person's eyes.

Bring your eyeglasses or contact lenses to your eye exam appointment. The eye doctor will want to make sure the prescription for your eyeglasses is the best one for you. You will need an up-to-date prescription along with the PD measurement to purchase prescription eyewear at any optical store after the exam. Minimal eye exams usually consist of direct ophthalmoscopy through an undilated pupil, as well as these eye tests:

Visual acuity is a vision test of the eye's ability to detect fine detail. It is the quantitative measure of the eye's ability to see an in-focus image at a certain distance. This eye test is what most people associate with an eye exam. It is usually performed using a projected eye chart to measure each eye's distance visual acuity and a small, hand-held acuity chart to measure each eye's near vision.

During this test, which is also known as a refraction, you look through a phoropter while shown a series of lens choices. The phoropter looks like a giant set of binoculars with various rotating lenses. You are asked which of the two lenses in each choice looks clearer.

Based on your answers, the optometrist or ophthalmologist will continue to fine-tune the lens power until reaching a final eyeglasses prescription. The refraction determines the level of hyperopia (farsightedness), myopia (nearsightedness), astigmatism, and presbyopia (ability to read) of the eyes.

Pupil function is an eye test that includes inspecting the pupils for equal size, regular shape, reactivity to light, and direct and consensual accommodation.

Extraocular muscle motility is an eye examination of the function of the eye muscles. A doctor observes the movement of the eyes in six specific directions.

Color blindness eye test detects hereditary color vision deficiencies, as well as other possible eye health problems that may affect your color vision.

The glaucoma test is conducted after your eyes are numbed with special eye drops. You stare straight ahead into the slit lamp while the optometrist or ophthalmologist uses an instrument called a tonometer to measure your eye pressure (IOP or intraocular pressure). Since there are no warning signs of glaucoma until a person already has significant vision loss, routine eye exams that include a glaucoma test are essential to rule out early signs of glaucoma and protect your eyesight.

Pupil dilation is the technique of using drops in the eyes to enlarge your pupils. Once the eyes are dilated (about 20 to 30 minutes after the drops are put in), the eye doctor uses various instruments to look inside the eyes. Because pupil dilation allows for the most thorough evaluation of the health of the inside of the eyes, it is very important for people with risk factors for eye disease to have this examination.

Visual field test measures peripheral (side) vision. This eye test is done to measure loss of vision from conditions such as stroke or glaucoma.

Besides these common vision tests performed during a standard comprehensive eye exam, an optometrist or ophthalmologist may recommend other, more specialized eye tests, if they feel it is warranted. Many eye diseases are asymptomatic (without symptoms or not having easily observed symptoms), which is why medical professionals recommend that all people, including children, should have periodic and thorough eye examinations as part of routine primary care. Early eye exams are important because children need visual skills for learning.

9

How to Buy Glasses Online

I have been in the online eyewear business for almost twenty years, since I founded Eyeglasses.com in 1999. I am not a licensed optician, but I employ opticians in the business, and I have unique experience in selling eyewear online. We take great care to listen to the comments of our customers, and we provide a high-touch, high-service business on the internet. Here are some of the insights I have learned through the years.

Buying eyeglasses online is not for everyone. In fact, only about 3 to 5% of the eyewear industry has moved online, compared to 15% for other fashion categories. Buying glasses online offers you more selection and at a lower price than at most optical stores. However—and that's why reading this guide will help you—buying online does require that you educate yourself first. You can choose between learning about eyewear and making your own decisions or paying an optical store employee to make most of your decisions.

Buying eyeglasses or sunglasses online offers a different package of products and services and a different eyewear experience altogether compared to shopping in a traditional optical store.

There are many online eyewear stores. Most online stores offer lower quality, cheap eyeglasses. Some online stores offer only high-quality eyeglasses frames, lenses, and services. Check the online reviews and make sure to do business with a well-recommended company.

Whether you actually buy online or not, you should use internet stores to check the prices that you are being quoted at the optical store. Find out the brand and model number of a frame you like and check the price online by searching for "Brandname Modelname eyeglasses" or, for example, "Gucci GU1234 eyeglasses." Then you can compare those prices with the price your optical store is quoting. If the price is significantly less online, then you can order the frame only from the online store and take it to the optical store to have lenses installed. This is the easiest way to use the internet for eyewear shopping.

If you don't know what model you want, at many websites you can order a few frames (without lenses), try them on at home, and return for a full refund.

4 STEPS TO ORDER FRAMES ONLINE WITH PRESCRIPTION LENSES

1. Get Your Prescription and Pupil Distance Measurement.

To order frames with lenses, start by getting your vision prescription that includes your PD—the pupil distance measurement. Most eye doctors will not measure your PD unless you ask, so be sure to ask for it and write it down on your prescription. The eye doctors assume that the optician filling the prescription will take that measurement. If that is not convenient, you can call the store that last made glasses for you; they should have your PD on file.

2. Choose Single-Vision, Progressive, or Bifocal Lenses.

If you want single-vision lenses, you can skip this step. If you want (and need) multifocal lenses (progressive, bifocal, or trifocal), then you must pay attention to the height of the lens in the frame that you choose.

Lens height is known as the B measurement. The B measurement must be at least 27 mm, but you should allow 30 mm or more for multifocal lenses. In other words, the lens must be high enough to accommodate the various corrections. A too-short lens will not work.

3. **Choose a Frame.**

Need help choosing a frame or finding the right size frame? Online resources are available to help you, or you can call online companies for more help. Experiment with frame search functions to look through the online inventory for frames with your specific needs, such as frame size, material, and shape. You might even try on glasses virtually if you upload a photo of yourself. Still not sure? Most online stores will allow you to order multiple frames without lenses and return them for a full refund.

4. **Add Lenses.**

Once you have chosen a frame, you can add lenses to it. For much more information on frames and lens options, see those specific sections in this guide.

HOW TO MAIL IN YOUR FRAMES FOR REPLACEMENT LENSES

Online and browsing pages of frames and still confused about which frames to select? Consider this: Why not reuse your current frames (if you love them) with your new prescription? You can now find websites on the internet that offer a replacement lens service. You mail in your eyeglasses frames, and they can install new lenses for you—this service is called replacement lenses.

Mail your frames in with your new prescription, your name and phone number, and any instructions you may have.

If you just want to redo your existing lenses (let's say they are scratched), you do not need to send in the prescription because the lab can read your prescription from your old lenses. You can mail in your glasses, and the lens laboratory can install new lenses. However, occasionally a frame will break during lens installation and the lab cannot be held responsible if this happens to your frame.

HOW TO GET THE MOST OUT OF YOUR VISION INSURANCE: THE OUT-OF-NETWORK BENEFIT

Most vision insurance plans have an out-of-network benefit. When you buy glasses online, you start at a much lower price than buying at an optical store. Then you send your invoice to the insurance company and they will send you a check for the out-of-network benefit. This benefit can range from $0 to $150. Read the section below on vision insurance for much more detailed information on this hidden benefit.

10

When Style Is Everything in Eyewear Fashion Trends

When considering different eyewear fashions, you might be intrigued by vintage looks or move toward a modern frame. Perhaps you prefer classic or sporty. And then, of course, you might spend time trying on frames made from different materials such as metal, titanium, acetate, plastic, wood, or mixes of these products. That wall of frames in the optical shop will display glasses in colors too. Which one to choose?

Eyewear fashion trends are not as distinct as clothing trends. You should choose your eyewear first for shape, then size, and then color, as these are the most noticeable attributes.

The shape of eyeglasses is a function of your face shape, as I discussed early on in this buying guide. For example, retro styles have larger, rounder shapes and leave a "classical" connotation about the wearer. Cat-eye shapes are edgier, as are small shapes. Rimless designs are more sophisticated.

In this context, when I refer to the size of a frame, I am talking about the thickness of it. Thicker, plastic frames are more noticeable, while thinner metal and rimless frames are less noticeable and therefore make less of a statement. Are you trying to project a statement with your eyewear, or blend in?

Color is the third most important attribute, because it depends on the shape and size of the frame. For example, if you are wearing thin, rimless frames, the color is very hard for other people to see, so it does not matter that much. But for large, thick plastic frames, color choice is important. Most often, color is chosen to blend into a person's facial coloring (skin, eye, hair). But some people like to use contrasting colors to make a bolder statement.

Layered plastics offer interesting color combinations

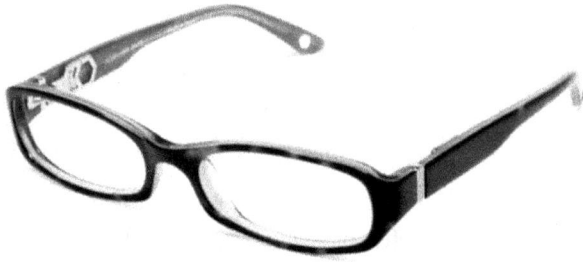

Ultimately when you put these three main characteristics together, you are looking to determine how you feel when wearing glasses with particular frames. If you don't feel really good in a frame, then keep looking.

WHAT'S IN AND WHAT'S OUT?

Vintage and retro have been popular in the media lately, but we see that trend waning as too many people looking for new fashions have gone there and are now beginning to swing back to something more edgy.

Solid colors used to dominate the scene, but now the trend is for more complicated layered colors. Smaller, boutique brands are coming back due to their beautiful coloring and chic-retro styling, which is a good bridge from the retro to the modern Parisian style.

The sheer and sleek look of the rimless styles continues to generate excitement, but more attention is being made to the temples of the rimless frames, which are not just small silver titanium strips anymore. Look for hi-tech plastics, plastics with a metal spine, and larger thicker temples made of plastic with the full variety of colors.

Retro styles are back

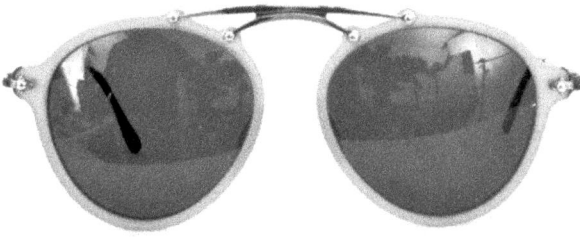

The size of a frame in relation to your head is a component of eyewear fashion trends. Too large frames are stylish in some seasons, especially in sunglasses, and for ladies it has the added bonus of making the head and face look smaller (shall I mention Audrey Hepburn here in *Breakfast at Tiffany's?*).

Conversely, some men like very small lenses in order to make their head and presence seem larger. And there are "right size" frames, which proportionately are neither too large nor too small, but have the advantage of looking well matched. Any of these combinations is a personal fashion choice, which will vary from person to person, and possibly from event to event. Unlike shoes or hats, there is no perfect size of glasses for any person.

11

How to Get the Most Out of Your Vision Insurance (Hint: It's Not Really Insurance)

If you have employer-provided vision insurance or have purchased such insurance on your own, it's important to know about your coverage.

Vision insurance benefits consist of two parts: the eye exam benefit and the eyewear benefit. Some optical providers are "in network" (meaning they are listed by your insurer as offering special pricing for you, the insured). Typically, these optical shops or providers sell frames and lenses at higher "sticker" prices and then apply the discount from the insurance plan. This system penalizes people without insurance, of course, because they will be asked to pay the full, marked-up pricing.

Fortunately, now there are high-quality eyewear providers who sell through internet stores at reasonable prices, not excessive markups.

Because most optical stores accept vision insurance for payment, they have increased all the prices of their prescription frames and lenses. Online stores do not inflate their prices, but they can't really help fit the frames to your face. The best way to use an insurance plan is to use the out-of-network benefit—*after you buy eyeglasses frames from an online store, where prices are the most competitive.*

So try this trick to use your vision insurance benefit but avoid paying too much.

- Step 1: Go to your in-network provider optical shop and choose a frame and get a price for glasses. You'll use this number for comparison.

- Step 2: Call your insurance company. Give them your plan number and your verifying information. Ask them to describe your out-of-network benefit for your plan. Ask for the information necessary to submit the out-of-network claim when you buy glasses from a provider who is not in the network.

- Step 3: Go online to an eyeglasses frame provider and price your glasses. (You may find the identical frame you priced at the optical shop.) Subtract from that your out-of-network benefit, and get your total price for glasses.

- Step 4: Compare that to the total price offered by your local optical store to determine the best value for you.

- Step 5: Take joy in knowing you are a smart shopper and have saved much more than this book cost you.

Here's an example of how to compare pricing using your out-of-network benefit: The store "sticker" price is $300 and you pay $136, so it looks as if you are saving $164—over 50%. This artificial increase in retail price makes people happy, and they continue to pay for the insurance plan. However, these inflated prices are deceiving when it comes to real savings. Take a closer look at all of the extra fees—copay, extras, plan fees—and you will see that your insurance "discount" is actually significantly more expensive than buying online and using your out-of-network benefit.

In this example, you are paying $206 to $352 in-network, and $129 to $209 out-of-network, a savings of $77 to $143. But many people have chosen to PAY for this insurance, which means you are paying another $150 per year on top of the cost for your eyewear!

How to Get the Most From Your Vision Benefit Plan In-Network vs. Out-of-Network		Typical Retail Price	Your Cost VSP In-Network	Your Cost Out-of-Network
	Frames	$300	$136	$200
	Lenses			
	SV Poly/UV/SC	$188	$45	$79
	Prog Poly/UV/SC	$350	$191	$159
	Crizal Advance No Glare	$130	$75	$89
	Copay		$25	
	OON Benefit			$85 - $150
	Your Cost	$488	$206	$194 - $129
		$650	$352	$274 - $209

*Plans and choice differ—Please ask your optical professional to give you a personal quote

VISION INSURANCE IS ESSENTIALLY A NATIONAL EYEWEAR TAX

Sold often as add-ons or options to employer health insurance plans, eyewear benefits are commonly misinterpreted as insurance. However, the terms are tightly limited and do not provide coverage for catastrophes. Premiums are typically quoted at $1 to $4 per week, and because that sounds like a small number, it is appealing to people. It has enticed more than 105 million people to add these programs to their coverage each year.

In some health plans, employees are paying for their eye exam twice. They get coverage both in their general health coverage and in the supplemental coverage that they add. This amounts to an additional $52 to $204 in annual costs, and a large percentage of customers fail to use their benefits during the year, which further increases profits for insurance companies.

Unfortunately, the human resources departments of large companies do not educate their employees about this problem and continue to offer vision "insurance" to employees as a so-called benefit.

Because so many people try to use their eyeglasses benefits when they shop for eyewear, the optical stores have raised their prices in order to accommodate the discounts that the plans offer. This has three effects:

- People without insurance are further penalized and forced to pay these higher prices.

- The national price of eyewear is inflated far above the factory price for the goods sold.

- Optical professionals, eyewear manufacturers, and insurance companies all benefit, and they have no incentive to change the system that penalizes all consumers.

The marketing of this "coverage" has led to a spike in the national price for eyewear. Insurance companies state that the average retail price for insurance covered eyewear is $414 to $513. To support these high costs, retailers must raise their prices to the detriment of those without insurance.

According to the Vision Council, 185 million people, or 75.5% of the adult population in the United States, require vision correction. Eyewear coverage imposes direct, definable price inflation and 48 million people who need glasses do not have them.

Eye care providers also are affected. The market forces them to increase their prices in order to discount them later, which simultaneously affects those without insurance. These providers are forced to spend less quality time with each patient to increase the quantity of patients to compete with the high insurance costs.

On average those with vision coverage pay $60 in premiums in addition to $90 in copays for a total of $150 and are limited to just one use of the benefits per year. However, a noninsured shopper can find $150 glasses through a quality retailer without wasting money on premiums.

WHAT CAN A SHOPPER DO?

Insurance companies hate it when you use the out-of-network benefit. When you stay in-network, it costs insurers nothing, because they have negotiated lower rates with eyecare professionals. When you use your out-of-network benefits, the insurance company has to write you a check.

For eyeglasses that are priced at about $150 or more, you can usually save money by getting several quotes for frames and lenses from optical stores, or online stores, getting the lowest price, and then submitting to your insurance company to get the benefit.

Get a clear description of what you want—brand, model number, color, and size of the frame, and exact description of the lens, and your prescription information. Submit all of this to eyewear stores online and in your town and get the best price.

If your best price is coming from an internet store, remember that they cannot provide fitting services. Some people prefer those fitting services, and you should consider how much more you are willing to pay to get those services from a local professional.

About the Author

Mark Agnew started Eyeglasses.com almost twenty years ago, in 1999. He had been working on Wall Street for the infamous investment bank Lehman Brothers. He worked in the volatile Emerging Markets area. One morning his boss told him the bank was getting out of that business, and Mark was asked to leave by the end of the day.

That wake-up call helped Mark reexamine what was important in life. He had been leaving the house early for the long commute and rarely saw his three young children or his wife. He decided that his family was more important.

He also realized that his vision was what distinguished him from most people—because in 1987 he had been mugged in the street and hit in the right eye with a stick. The attack caused blindness in his eye and left it with a cloudy color that looked like a cataract. Not only was he blinded, he was left with a visual distinction that every person he meets notices immediately. The injury was both a visual impairment and a cosmetic challenge.

He wanted to help other people with their vision and also to help them look their best. And that epiphany in the aftermath of losing his Wall Street job was the answer: eyeglasses. Mark bought the website Eyeglasses.com during the early days of the internet and launched his company.

Eyeglasses.com has sold over 1 million glasses to people over the internet. But it was a struggle in the beginning and continues to be a struggle, because optical stores complained bitterly to the suppliers to stop supplying online stores. Opticians and optometrists continue to tell customers that buying online is for idiots and morons. Suppliers continue to restrict online sales either outright, or by enforcing "suggested retail prices." Eyeglasses.com is the classic industry disrupter because Mark's company offers education, choice, and rational pricing.